GOOD DRU

CONTENTS

I. Introduction

II. The Limitations of Western Medicine

III. Alternatives to Western Medicine

IV. Seven Strategies of Wholesome Living

    1. sound nutrition
    2. adequate exercise
    3. adequate rest
    4. relaxation
    5. cleanliness
    6. an occasional fast
    7. a positive outlook

V. Nothing to Lose but Much to Gain

VI. Appendix

VII. Bibliography

I

INTRODUCTION

For many people the first step towards disease is the trip to the doctor's office.

There is a desperate need for a book like GOOD HEALTH WITHOUT DRUGS OR DOCTORS, in the developed parts of the world as well as in developing countries. With Western medicine, the world – both the developed and the developing parts of it -- has acquired a system of health care it can ill afford and which does little good. The big multi-national drug companies are the driving force behind that medical system. But their prime concern is profits, not health. Their interests, in fact, run counter to a sensible health care system: they want to sell more, and more expensive, drugs whereas a sane health care system would be vitally interested in reducing to a minimum the incidence of disease, thereby reducing to a minimum the need for drugs.

Western Medicine, as GOOD HEALTH WITHOUT DRUGS OR DOCTORS will point out, fails people everywhere. It looks for the causes of disease in forces largely beyond the control of the individual -- germs, environmental poisons, hereditary factors, etc. It takes disease for granted and accordingly places its bets on the corrective therapies --- drugs, surgery and radiation. But these corrective therapies do not build or even maintain health. At best they alleviate the symptoms; at worst they make the sick sicker. Western Medicine is not interested in building health. There is no money to be made from healthy people. Western Medicine is big business that benefits nothing so much as itself.

The major alternative, Naturopathic Medicine, looks for the causes of disease in faulty living habits. It believes that there would be very little illness if people lived right. Naturopathic Medicine considers it its main task to teach people how to live so that eventually they won't need drugs or doctors. That's no faddist pipe dream but an objective that can be achieved. Healthy people anywhere, individuals or groups like the Hunza, owe their good health not to the ministrations of Western Medicine but to a wholesome lifestyle. Healthy people, by and large, do not consume drugs. It is the sick who do, and often the drugs make them sicker.

From a naturopathic point of view, living so that one won't get sick means practicing the seven strategies of wholesome living discussed in some detail in Chapter IV -- sound nutrition, adequate exercise, adequate rest, relaxation, cleanliness, an occasional fast and a positive outlook. These strategies can be relied on to build health and to maintain it far into old age. These same strategies can be relied on to restore health that has broken down. Ultimately man's best doctor is his own body. If the naturopathic philosophy of health is put into practice, the rewards will be tremendous. For the individual it will mean freedom from illness and freedom from the fear of illness; for society it will mean reducing health care costs to a bare minimum and freeing for use in other areas the vast financial and human resources now tied up in health care. The author himself is living proof that this is possible. Though he is pushing 80, he is superbly healthy and fit. He is on no drugs and hasn't been on any drugs for more than four decades. Wouldn't you like to be like him?

An eighth strategy might have been added – stay away from drugs and doctors. But that's the theme of the whole book. And, if you practice all the other strategies as discussed in the book, you will not need drugs or doctors anyway.

II

THE LIMITATIONS OF WESTERN MEDICINE

My body, with the help of the good Lord, heals itself but my doctor claims the fee.
(G.B. Shaw)

It is not difficult to find population groups that do not use western drugs and yet are as healthy as, if not healthier than, those who do. The Hunza, a small nation in northern Pakistan, are such a group, and their good health is proverbial. Western medical investigators, who went to Hunzaland to find out just what it was that accounted for the enviable good health of the Hunza, could hardly believe the evidence of their senses: a set of people generally so healthy that they needed neither drugs nor doctors, many of them old beyond what we think possible and still in vigorous good health, some as old as 100 and still working in their fields. And virtually no medical services in our sense, just a lifestyle that makes and keeps them healthy.

The Christian Science people, reject western drugs altogether and rely instead on a healthy lifestyle and on spiritual means of healing. If good health depended mainly on the use of drugs, those Christian Scientists should be among the sickest people in the world. Not so, say American insurance companies, who should know. They do not consider Christian Scientists worse insurance risks than anyone else in the USA.

One could name other sets of people, past and present, who achieved good health without western drugs, such as the Eskimos of northern Canada and Alaska, or the Indians of the Vilcabamba area in Ecuador. As for the Eskimos, early explorers sent home glowing reports about their good health. Unfortunately that wonderful good health has been disappearing fast, in spite of -- perhaps because of -- their exposure to white man's supposedly superior ways of living.

Medical literature records a number of situations where doctors went on strike. Contrary to expectations, the people thus deprived of their doctors' services did not seem any the worse for it. Let us look at one such situation. In 1972, the doctors of Los Angeles County in California withheld their services from all but emergency cases. When the strike was over and investigators went in to assess the damage, they discovered, much to their surprise, that there **had been no damage**. Most people had suffered little, if any, inconvenience during the slow-down. And the investigators discovered something even more surprising -- that the death rate had actually gone down in the county while the doctors were off the job. The investigators attributed the drop in the death rate to fewer drugs and less surgery.

Much the same happened in Israel in 1973, as Dr. Mercola tells us. The doctors of Israel went on strike for a month and the death rate dropped by 50 per cent. The full story is here:

lib.store.yahoo.net/lib/realityzone/UFNDrsstrikefewerdie.htm

If it seems possible to be healthy without western drugs, do the drugs at least make healthy those who use them? Well, if it is *making healthy* in the sense an antibiotic cures an infection, some drugs do make healthy. If, however, it is *making healthy* in the sense a wholesome diet and exercise make healthy, no drugs make anyone healthy. Drugs do not build health. At best they take care of the symptoms. But a great many drugs in our pharmacies don't even do that: they don't do what they are supposed to do but do things they are **not** supposed to do; that is, they do not cure but have nasty side effects. At worst, they make people sicker. Some of them actually kill. In areas of the world where western drugs are commonly used, those people who are healthy are so not because of drugs but because of a wholesome way of living coupled perhaps with inherited good genes. They are in fact the ones who use drugs very seldom, if at all. It is the sick who consume the drugs. And all-too frequently the drugs make them sicker.

Apart from their toxic side effects, drugs can harm patients in ways that easily escape notice: by alleviating the symptoms of an illness without effecting a cure of the illness itself, they can give the patient a false sense of well-being, prompting him to ignore the body's warning signals and to persist in his health-destroying living habits -- smoking, drinking, a faulty diet, no exercise, not enough rest, etc. -- something that could seriously aggravate his condition.

The medications used to fight the common cold may serve to illustrate the point. Though scores of anti-cold drugs are available, both over the counter and on prescription, there is not a single one of which it could be said with certainty that it does anything to cure a cold. Every honest doctor will tell you so. Yet lots of them are prescribed and lots more are bought over the counter. What they do is alleviate the nasty symptoms of a cold -- the headache, the muscle pains which frequently accompany a cold, the feeling of weakness, the stuffy nose, etc. They accomplish this mainly by means of painkillers and stimulants. The patient takes one or two of them and presto he feels better: pain gone, that feeling of weakness gone, depression lifting. Why stay in bed? He gets up and resumes his routine of frantic activity which was instrumental in causing the cold in the first place, instead of doing what his body prompts him to do -- rest, to give it a better chance really to heal itself. Things get worse rather than better. Having, moreover, to battle the toxins that come with the drugs, it takes the body longer to cure the cold than it would have taken without the drugs. Is it any wonder that some colds seem to drag on forever?

Virtually all drugs are dangerous, whether they do any good or not. Even a safe drug like aspirin can have adverse side effects for some people. But don't expect the maker of a drug -- or the doctor who prescribes it -- to tell you: "This drug is dangerous. There is evidence that it has killed people. It may kill you. If you want to use it, go ahead; but you should be aware of the risks."

Doctors themselves often do not know how dangerous a given drug may be. Drug companies do, but they won't tell unless they are compelled to tell by court rulings. Do you find this hard to believe? Well, let's look at some real evidence.

There is the story of Butazolidin, a popular drug used in the treatment of arthritis and rheumatism. Prior to 1982, its maker, the Swiss multinational giant Ciba Geigy, had admitted that the drug was not altogether safe, had admitted that there could be such side effects as internal bleeding, skin problems and hematological changes. The company had even owned up to some 76 deaths attributed to the drug between 1952 and 1982. Then a Swedish doctor produced evidence in court that Ciba Geigy had much more damning information hidden away in secret company files; to wit, documentation of a total of 701 Butazolidin deaths, almost ten times as many as they had admitted.

The story of Tanderil, another anti-rheumatism drug, is similar. While its maker, the same Ciba Geigy, had admitted 70 deaths for the time between 1960 and 1982, there was evidence of 329 Tanderil deaths locked away in secret files at company headquarters.

And there is the story of Mexaform, a drug once widely used in the treatment of diarrhea. The same Swedish doctor, who took on Ciba over Butazolidin and Tanderil, had been instrumental in exposing the Mexaform scandal a year or two earlier. Among the most frequent side effects of the drug were damage to the optic nerve, peripheral neuropathy (tingling sensation of the skin, a feeling as if ants were crawling over the skin), various forms of paralysis, and death. In Japan alone, 11,000 cases of Mexaform damage were confirmed by the Ministry of Health. Loss of sight was the most frequently cited complication. One thousand deaths were attributed to the drug.

After such disclosures, one would expect these drugs to be discontinued at once. Not so. What often happens is that the maker of an incriminated drug sheds a few crocodile tears in public. Behind the scenes he plays a delaying game -- drags the issue through the courts, from appeal to appeal, until the stockpiles of the drug have been sold. Then he agrees to withdraw it from the market. The big pharmaceutical companies sell drugs that have been shown to maim and kill as long as they can hope to get away with it. And, if massive pressure of public indignation and court orders should compel them to withdraw certain drugs from the markets of the developed countries, there is still the vast market of the developing countries to keep dumping those drugs on until supplies are exhausted. Nobody is likely to make much noise about side effects there.

Take Mexaform again. It had been banned in most developed countries by the end of 1984. According to the "Tagesanzeiger," a leading Swiss paper (Dec. 4, 1984), Ciba had agreed to withdraw the drug completely early in 1985, sooner than originally agreed on. Yet a year later (December 1985), I found the drug on the shelves of several pharmacies of Maiduguri, a city in Northern Nigeria. The salesmen there were not aware that the drug had been banned. Two of the pharmacies I checked, by the way, also had both Butazolidin and Tanderil in stock. As late as 1986, a professor of Medicine at the Maiduguri University Teaching Hospital prescribed Mexaform.

Are you shocked to learn that the big pharma-companies are not the selfless benefactors of mankind they would like us to believe they are? For your own good, you should understand that their prime concern is profit, not health. They are in business to make money, not to help humanity. In fact, as I indicated above, the interests of the big pharma-companies actually run counter to a rational health care system: the pharma-industry wants to sell more, and more expensive, drugs, but a sane health care scheme would be vitally interested in reducing to a minimum the incidence of disease, thereby reducing to a minimum the need for drugs.

Of the three basic types of therapy practiced by Western Medicine -- drug therapy, surgery, radiotherapy -- drugs are by far the most important one. Drugs are what most patients get from the practitioners of Western Medicine. In fact, drugs are so much taken for granted that most patients would feel disappointed if they were dismissed from a doctor's office without a prescription. Yet, as I pointed out above, drugs do not build health. At best they alleviate the symptoms; at worst they make the sick sicker.

What I have said about drugs applies largely to the other two pillars of Western Medicine -- surgery and radiotherapy. Neither of them builds health. At best they patch up health that has broken down. At worst they do harm. And both would be largely unnecessary if people lived the way they should live.

Yet this Western Medicine has all but conquered the world . In most developed countries it has contrived to eliminate virtually all competition from alternate health care systems and has become *the* system. Even in developing countries it has in large measure displaced native systems of health care. In most of them it has, in fact, become the official system of health care. It would, however be wrong to attribute this global spread of Western Medicine primarily to its effectiveness as a health care scheme. Its success is rather due to the business acumen of its representatives.

Western Medicine has no doubt done some good, but it has not done nearly as much good as medical propaganda would have us believe. It probably deserves little credit for the spectacular rise in life expectancy, which most of the developed countries experienced between the middle of the 19th and the middle of the 20th century. Around 1850, a newborn baby could look forward to a life expectancy of about forty years. A hundred years later, the average life expectancy in most of the developed world had risen to around seventy years. But the figures are deceptive.

It is important to note that most of the gains in longevity were due to the prevention of mortality at young ages -- at childbirth, in infancy and in early childhood -- where infectious diseases had been taking a heavy toll. But infectious diseases were conquered less through vaccinations and modern miracle drugs than through improvements in hygiene and nutrition. If a baby born today can expect to live about thirty years longer than one born a hundred years earlier, very little gain has been made in the life expectancy of people past the mid-mark of life. Today a fifty-year-old man can expect to live all of two years longer than he could have a hundred years ago.

Meanwhile, degenerative diseases -- heart disease, diabetes, arthritis, ulcers, cancer, etc. -- have increased at an alarming rate in the Western World. A hundred years ago, only about one in ten deaths was attributable to degenerative diseases. Today degenerative diseases claim more than half of all deaths. And ***visavis*** degenerative diseases, Western Medicine is singularly helpless. The best it has to offer is patchwork, and alleviation of the symptoms. It has no cures. And that is not surprising. Degenerative diseases are largely the cumulative effect of years of faulty living. The ministrations of Western Medicine cannot take the place of a healthful lifestyle. Western Medicine is pretty good at surgery where surgery is indicated -- in accidents, for instance; and it can generally be trusted to do a good job of combating infections by means of antibiotics or the sulfa drugs. But the victim of arthritis or of cancer is probably well advised to go to an alternative practitioner rather than to a practitioner of Western Medicine.

Even infectious diseases can have the rug pulled out from under them by natural means. Bugs of every description thrive in a setting where the pH factor is below 7; i.e. on the acidic side of the spectrum. If the pH is above 7; that is, if it is on the alkaline side of the scale, disease-causing germs have no chance. Neither, by the way, does cancer. For a heart-warming story of a man who used baking soda to cure himself of prostate cancer that had already metastasized to his bones go to <http://phkillscancer.com/> He used baking soda to raise his pH factor till it was above 7; that is alkaline. In an alkaline environment, it seems, cancer has no chance. Nor is this an isolated case. Don't believe me? Just do a search for "Baking soda against cancer."

If Western Medicine does not do nearly as much good as it would have us believe, it can take credit for doing a lot of harm. It has done and continues to do harm mainly in two ways -- it imparts a kind of health education that is, by and large, counterproductive and it often harms the patient through the very therapies that are supposed to cure him.

One of the worst things Western Medicine has done to us is that it has robbed us of our faith in the healing powers of our own bodies and given us instead something that amounts to an obsession with medication. For the least little thing we run to doctors' offices, where we expect to be treated to some form of therapy -- a pill, a needle, a bit of infra-red or ultraviolet or X-ray therapy, perhaps even surgery. Owing to the brainwashing we have been subjected to at the hands of Western Medicine, we have all but forgotten the basic truth -- a very heartening truth, by the way -- that the human body is altogether capable of dealing with most of the everyday ills which most of us develop every now and then How would humanity have survived the millennia if this were not so? Humanity has existed for millions of years while Western Medicine as we know it is barely a century old.

Most of the common ills that bring people to doctors' offices -- influenza, a cold, sore tonsils, a touch of fever, a touch of diarrhea -- are "self-limiting"; that is, they run their course, medication or no medication, from an initial phase characterized by a general feeling of malaise, to the climax of a healing crisis and a gradual return to normal. The doctors of yesteryear used to tell their patients, "A cold takes seven days if you treat it and a week if you don't treat it." Today's doctors know that too, but they are not going to tell a patient, "Nothing wrong with you. You have abused your body in one way or other, and it is letting you know. What you need is not a doctor but a little extra Vitamin C and D and a few days of rest. Just go home, skip a meal or two and rest. In a few days you will be as good as new. There is really nothing I can do for you." This sort of honesty would shake the patient's faith in the doctor's omniscience and it would be bad for business.

What happens quite often is that the patient does not actually see his doctor at the first sign of an illness. He waits a while, hoping against hope that the illness will go away. It would too, if only he waited long enough. For, unbeknownst to him, his body initiates action at once: it takes his appetite away so that he will eat less, perhaps fast altogether;

it makes him feel weak so as to impel him to rest; it generates a fever, one of the most important weapons in the fight against infections; it makes him sweat in order to expedite the elimination of metabolic waste; it makes him feel thirsty so that he will take in extra fluid, etc. Thanks to these and other measures, healing is initiated at once. But it takes time.

The patient however cannot wait, mainly because he has no faith in the healing powers of his body. Medical propaganda has taken that faith from him and given him instead the dubious certainty that he can hope to get well only if he takes some medication or other. So he rushes to the doctor's office. Nothing much happens there. He hardly gets a chance to recite his catalogue of complaints, for Doc's a terribly busy man. In no time at all, Mr. Patient finds himself back in the waiting room. But there is a difference: he has a prescription in his hand. Thank God for that! Off he goes to the pharmacy, where he obtains several kinds of pills, one to be taken in the morning, and another to be taken every four hours. Even before he crawls into bed that night he feels better. Most of his aches and pains seem to have vanished. When the alarm clock tolls him back to reality in the morning, he feels almost himself again. Wonderful stuff, those pills! Wonderful chap, that doctor! Really knows what he's doing.

Mr. Patient is not likely ever to know that it was not the pills that cured him but his own body. When he appeared at the doctor's office, his body had been busy healing itself for several days; in fact, it had almost finished doing so -- it had reached the healing crisis, the point where an illness is said to peak and after which there is a dramatic change for the better. His recovery had been only one night away. But because he had swallowed the pills, he attributed his improvement to the pills. ***Post hoc, ergo propter hoc.***

If doctors don't seem eager to undeceive patients about drugs, the big drug companies are even less so. Drugs are big business. The world over, humanity probably spends close to half a trillion dollars on drugs, and the pharma-industry spends untold millions of dollars annually on advertising designed to make people buy even more drugs.

And some of the advertising is downright fraudulent. If you click **http://www.usatoday.com/money/industries/health/2009-09-02-pfizer-fine_N.htm** you'll learn that very recently pharma giant Pfizer, was fined 2.3 billion dollars "in the largest health care fraud settlement in history."

Western Medicine shows very little, if any, interest in genuine disease prevention. There is no money in prevention, but there is lots of money to be made from creating and perpetuating the illusion that good health can be had only from Western Medicine, in particular from drugs.

Western Medicine has no use for the notion that, with very few exceptions, disease is the result of faulty living, and that in most cases the most effective therapy would be for the patient to find out what is faulty about his living habits and to correct them. Nothing arouses the ire of Western Medicine more surely than to contend that there would be very little illness if people lived right. For, if this suggestion were taken seriously, a big part of Western Medicine would eventually be done out of business. But the last thing big business wants is to see itself done out of business.

Western Medicine then does harm by robbing man of his faith in the healing power of his body and creating instead the illusion that good health can be had only from Western Medicine. *Iatrogenic disease* is a term denoting another kind of harm done by Western Medicine. Literally it means harm done by the doctor. Hippocrates, the famous physician of ancient Greece, believed that a doctor's first concern had to be not to do harm. This is reflected in the Hippocratic Oath, which Western Medicine carries on its banner. In the practice of Western Medicine, alas, this oath is often violated.

Bittere Pillen (Nutzen und Risiken der Arzneimittel – Bitter Pills, Usefulness and Risks of Medical Drugs.) reports that in England roughly one in twelve patients admitted to hospital is admitted owing to the side effects of drugs. Worse, of patients already in hospital, one in ten suffers serious harm from drugs (s)he is given there. These figures are, if anything, low because it is extremely difficult to assess long-term damage done by drugs. Even short-term damage all-too frequently goes unidentified, if not unnoticed. If a patient suffers from adverse side effects of a drug, both he and the doctor are likely to regard them as a worsening of his condition rather than as effects of therapy -- the patient, because he doesn't know any better; the doctor, because he'd rather not admit that the drug(s) made the patient sicker.

Surveys done in several German hospitals showed that as many as 20% of all hospital patients can expect to suffer serious harm from drugs administered there.

Certain medical fads come under the heading of iatrogenic disease. A few decades ago, lots of people lost their teeth owing to a medical fad prevalent at the time which held that one of the causes of rheumatism and arthritis was infected teeth. Hundreds of thousands of people became the victims of another medical fad. They lost their tonsils because Western Medicine believed that infected tonsils were the cause of an assortment of illnesses. Today at least some western practitioners have come to understand that infected tonsils are not so much a cause as a symptom – a symptom of an organism overloaded with the toxins of accumulated metabolic waste. The cure – to detoxify the organism, not to cut out the tonsils.

I remember a cartoon which showed an American doctor looking into a patient's mouth. The caption -- "I see, you still have your tonsils. While we have you here, we might as well take them out too." Not so long ago, appendectomy -- the surgical removal of the appendix -- ran a close second to tonsillectomy. In some circles it was sarcastically referred to as bread-and-butter surgery. Surgical removal of the gall bladder, largely unnecessary, is bread-and-butter surgery still widely practiced today.

Wherever Western Medicine "operates," but especially in the USA, lots of people get treated to unnecessary surgery every year. And lots of people die from it. That's iatrogenic disease at its worst.

You may find it hard to believe that there should be such a thing as unnecessary surgery on a large scale. Well, in Western Medicine, surgery is probably the most prestigious, quite certainly one of the most lucrative branches of medical specialization. That's why lots of ambitious medical students want to get into surgery. The result is a surplus of surgeons. But those surgeons don't want to be idle, not after all the time and money they have invested in becoming surgeons. So they operate. The patient may not need the operation, but the surgeon does. The more operations, the more money for the surgeon.

In countries -- most third-world countries and some of the developed countries -- where surgeons are salaried professionals, not professional businessmen, there is little temptation to carry out unnecessary operations and little risk for a patient to become the victim of an unnecessary operation.

In America, one of the big money-makers for surgeons is hysterectomy, the surgical removal of the womb and the ovaries. It used to be performed when there was a confirmed diagnosis of uterine cancer. But there obviously were not enough cases of uterine cancer to go around. So American surgeons came up with the idea of the ***prophylactic hysterectomy***. Many of them actually advise women past child-bearing age to submit to hysterectomy as a means of preventing cancer of the uterus and/or of the ovaries, even though those organs are perfectly healthy. What a lucrative field! Lucky American women, to have such surgeons looking after them! I wonder how those hundreds of millions of women the world over, who don't have access to American medical care, are going to make it through the second half of life with their *uteri* and their ovaries still in their appointed places. Want to know about possible side effects of hysterectomy, whether it is necessary or not? Well, here are some of them: precipitating the mid-life crisis, tripling the risk of heart attacks, upsetting the delicate balance of the endocrine glands, depression, etc. No doubt, however, the benefits of the procedure outweigh the harmful side effects -- the *financial* benefits of the hysterectomising surgeons, that is.

Delivery by Caesarean is a popular medical procedure in the USA. I remember an article in a Nigerian paper, which warned well-to-do Nigerian women to think twice about having their babies in the USA, for there they would be as likely as not to have them by Caesarean. Much more money to be made from a Caesarean delivery than from a conventional one. Besides, an ordinary delivery can happen at any time, even in the middle of the night, while a delivery by Caesarean can be planned so that it does not inconvenience the obstetrician.

A third surgical procedure of comparable magnitude is about to take its place beside hysterectomy and the Caesarean -- mastectomy, or the removal of breasts, for women past child-bearing or for women who don't want children. The reason? Well, to protect them against breast cancer. Lucky American women to have such surgeons looking after them! Think of the hundreds of millions of women in other parts of the world who have to go through the later parts of their lives with their breasts where nature put them!

III

IF NOT WESTERN MEDICINE, WHAT ALTERNATIVE?

There is wide-spread disenchantment with Western Medicine in the West. More and more people look for alternatives, especially those who have been treated by practitioners of Western Medicine, often for years, with little or no success, those whom Western Medicine left worse off than they had been before treatment. More and more people are placing their bets on a change of lifestyle -- living so that they won't get sick in the first place, living so that they won't need the ministrations of Western Medicine.

I myself subscribed to Western Medicine without reservations for the first three and a half decades of my life. Then, some forty-five years ago, I had my Road-to-Damascus experience. A librarian friend of mine pushed Adele Davis's LET'S EAT RIGHT TO KEEP FIT into my hand and told me to read it. That book made all the difference. Long before I had finished it, my vision began to clear. I began to understand that good health is not something I could get from a doctor but something I would have to work for myself.

Fired by the new understanding, I got myself started on a general program of self-education in matters of fitness and health, and I set out to survey the medical scene for alternatives to Western Medicine. Naturopathy, Hydrotherapy, Chiropractic, Herbalism, Homeopathy, Phytotherapy -- after a good look at all of them I was convinced that Naturopathic Medicine held more promise than any other system, Western Medicine included. So I decided to study Naturopathic Medicine myself, and eventually I obtained an N.D., the naturopathic equivalent of an M.D. I did not get to practice Naturopathy, except for a little freelancing here and there, but the knowledge I gained has stood me in good stead personally. For more than four decades I have lived the naturopathic way. In all that time I have had no need of doctors or drugs, and I have felt superbly healthy. And that in environments as different one from the other as mid-latitude Halifax in Eastern Canada, tropical Maiduguri in sub-Saharan Africa, the Philippines and Jeddah on the Red Sea coast of Saudi Arabia.

However, though I did not get to practice Naturopathy, I am still glad that I studied that line of medicine for all it has done for me and some people close to me. The naturopathic way of life is the best of health-insurance schemes. It is something one can comfortably live and confidently grow old with. Want to join me in having a closer look?

Naturopathic Medicine puts the responsibility for health squarely on the individual's shoulders. It holds that, except in very exceptional cases, good health is not a matter of genetic accident, not something bestowed on some and withheld from others by capricious gods, not something to be obtained from even the most spectacular medical procedures -- kidney dialysis, open-heart surgery, organ transplants, etc. Good health, Naturopathic Medicine holds, is each man's own responsibility, his own to make or to mar.

The human body is a marvelous piece of biological engineering. By a wisdom which all the scientific posturing of man cannot begin to fathom, it contrives to build itself in all its complexity from two tiny cells met in conception. It knows how to maintain itself from day today. Doesn't need a doctor or drugs for all that. And, if given half a chance, that same body can repair itself if something should go wrong. Ultimately no doctor can cure you. Your body has to do the curing. The best a good doctor can do is to assist your body in curing itself. All-too frequently doctors get in the way with medications that are either not needed or the wrong ones, and the body has to cure itself in spite of their ministrations. Luckily each of us can count, at all times, on the services of this best of doctors, his own body.

The day when I understood this basic and most heartening truth stands out as a red-letter day in my private calendar. I felt a tremendous sense of relief, a sense of liberation. Gone was that insidious fear of sickness and of death resulting from sickness. Where before I had felt touches of panic when the first signs of illness appeared, I now viewed such things as a headache, a fever, a cough, a touch of diarrhea as mere signals which my body sent me to let me know that I was on the wrong track. In the old system of beliefs, I would have regarded them as illnesses to be treated. I would have opted for the headache pill, the antipyretic, the cough syrup, the antibiotic. Now I knew that all I had to do was to get back on track. My body would do the rest. Just what being on track or getting back on track means in the present context will be explained in detail in the next chapter -- the chapter dealing with the seven basic naturopathic strategies of building health.

But, before I go any further, I'd like to offer a definition of *health*. To the orthodox medical establishment health is primarily the absence of disease and the measuring up to certain "normal" values in certain checks and on certain tests -- blood pressure, heart rate, hemoglobin count, cholesterol level, etc. However, there are among the millions of people who frequent the offices of western doctors countless thousands who do not feel their state of health is what it should and might be though they check out as "normal" in every way. Eventually one of two things is likely to happen to them. Either they are told that there is nothing wrong with them, that the aches and pains they feel are merely "psychosomatic." Nothing more Family Doctor can do for them. They had better see a specialist, that is a psychiatrist. Or the family doctor decides to treat the symptoms. Morbid state of listlessness? Chronic lack of energy? No problem. The doctor prescribes his favorite brand of stimulant and, at least for a while, the patient is satisfied and seemingly better. State of anxiety, mental or emotional problems? Doc prescribes his favorite line of tranquilizers.

The trouble with most of the conventional medical checks and tests is that the values regarded as normal are not normal so much as <u>average</u> -- average in terms of samples obtained from population groups that are a long way from being healthy. Take heart rate for example. The medical establishment accepts as normal in an adult a resting heart rate of 65 to 85. But that is high. A genuinely healthy adult, one whose cardiovascular system is in good shape thanks to regular aerobic exercise, is likely to have a resting heart rate that is considerably lower than 65; lower, that is, than what the establishment considers the low end of normal. The heart rate of a healthy athlete may be as low as 30 beats per minute. A <u>normal</u> heart rate of 65 to 85 is not normal; it rather represents an average of a population group that is out of shape. Similar cases could be made for the normal values of many of the medical checks and tests, which the medical establishment makes so much of.

What Western Medicine considers HEALTH is not genuine HEALTH, at least not in the eyes of a naturopath. For the naturopath, genuine health also starts with the absence of disease, such conditions as acne, allergies, overweight and bad breath included. Someone with a face full of acne cannot be considered genuinely healthy though all his checks and tests be normal. Nor can he whose weight is more than 10 % above what would be his ideal weight. But there is more to genuine good health than the absence of disease. He who would qualify as genuinely healthy functions well on all levels-- the physical, the physiological, the psychological and the philosophical levels. He has more than enough energy to cope with the exigencies of ordinary living and quite enough to cope with the occasional crisis. Young or old, he climbs several flights of stairs without gasping for breath. His senses are acute. No need for glasses or hearing aids. His breath is sweet. He has at least one bowel movement a day, ideally one after each meal. His digestive system works so smoothly that he seldom, if ever, becomes aware of it. He rarely breaks wind because there is no flatulence; and if he does, there is no foul odor. His sweat does not smell, so there is no need for deodorants. On the psychological level he has no trouble coping with the ordinary stresses of life, and he has at his disposal enough psychic energy to deal with an emergency now and then. No need for uppers or downers, whether they be prescribed as drugs by the medical establishment or pushed by the corporate establishment as coffee, sugar, alcohol or nicotine. On the spiritual level, he has a healthy optimism and he is at peace with himself and his world.

A COMPARISON AND CONTRAST

Let us look at Naturopathy first. It looks for the causes of disease primarily in the individual's lifestyle. If people lived right, the naturopath believes, they would cope well with what Western Medicine considers the causes of disease and there would be very little illness in the world. In other words, Naturopathy puts the responsibility for health squarely on the individual's showlders.

The naturopath regards germs as secondary, not as primary causes of disease. He considers germs the scavengers of diseased tissue, healthy tissue being largely immune to them. As for the degenerative diseases, Naturopathy offers cures where Western Medicine has no more than symptomatic relief to offer. Though doctors may not know the causes of certain diseases, Doctor Body knows. And it knows how to remedy them if given a chance.

Naturopathic Medicine leaves diagnosis largely to the body. This practice has two important advantages -- one, that the body's diagnostic efforts are cheap; two, that they are very reliable. Body is virtually never wrong. No risk therefore of wrong treatment or iatrogenic disease. In Naturopathic Medicine there is basically only one disease entity -- an organism off track owing to faulty living, even though the external manifestations of disease differ greatly from individual to individual. And there is basically only one course of action -- to get the organism back on track by correcting the faulty living habits. No harm can come of that.

Naturopathic Medicine is primarily concerned with health. It considers this its main mission – to teach people how to live so that they won't need doctors or drugs. That's no faddist pipe dream but a very real possibility. From a naturopathic point of view, an ideal patient is well-informed and prepared to assume full responsibility for his own health. Western Medicine, on the contrary, does not want informed patients. For most western practitioners a good patient is one who does not presume to know much about health care in general or his particular problem(s), and who does obediently, no questions asked, what Doc tells him to do.

Naturopathic Medicine addresses itself to the real causes of disease -- faulty living habits. By helping a patient correct the faults in his living habits, it helps him genuinely to regain his health. No risk though that naturopathy would run out of patients in the foreseeable future.

Since most naturopaths practice what they preach, they are, by and large, a healthy lot. Just what the naturopathic way of life is will be explained in the next chapter. As you will see, there is nothing peculiar about it. It simply means living according to the laws of nature, the way we should be living anyway. I myself have been living that way for four decades; and, though I am crowding eighty, I don't know what it means to sick. I hope to live to at least a hundred and to stay healthy all the way. A naturopathic lifestyle is more likely than any other lifestyle I know to get me there.

Now for a glance at Western or Mainstream Medicine, which views disease as the result of either errors in an individual's genetic make-up or of forces outside him and generally beyond his control -- germs, environmental poisons, environmental stresses, etc. Another category of diseases -- those ascribed to causes unknown such as arthritis, diabetes, cancer, allergies and high blood pressure – coincides roughly with what is commonly referred to as degenerative diseases. Western Medicine is singularly helpless *vis a vis* this kind of disease. Palliative treatment is all it has to offer, perhaps "control" of the disease, but no cure.

In Western Medicine it is terribly important to arrive at a diagnosis -- to stick a label on a disease, as it were. The diagnosis of course determines the therapy. But in the practice of Western Medicine, diagnosis is not nearly as reliable as it is made out to be. Go to five different doctors and get five different diagnoses for the same complaint. But, if the diagnosis is wrong, the treatment is bound to be wrong too, sometimes with dreadful consequences.

Too busy diagnosing separate disease entities and patching up health that has broken down, Western Medicine does not have time for or interest in building health. Moreover, even if the interest were there, most western practitioners could do very little to promote health because that's not part of their training. In their medical schools they learn all about diseases but very little about health. Besides, the notion of building health runs counter to the very nature of Western Medicine *qua* big business: by building health it would put large parts of itself out of business.

Western Medicine addresses itself mainly to the symptoms of disease. Even if it is apparently successful in that the symptoms disappear, the patient is bound to get sick again because nothing is done to remove the real cause of disease – faulty living habits. This way Western Medicine will never run out of patients.

Western physicians are their own most unfortunate patients. They suffer as much from degenerative diseases and from deficiency diseases as their patients -- they die of diseases of the heart and of the blood vessels; they have pyorrhea and tooth decay; they are crippled by arthritis and neuritis; they have stomach ulcers and cancer. Not a few of them smoke, not a few of them are alcoholics or even drug addicts. And most of these problems could be prevented if Western Medicine showed a little less interest in disease and a little more interest in health. It is significant that the life expectancy of Western doctors is rather lower than the general life expectancy.

Western Medicine has made much noise about "preventive medicine" of late, but the term does not mean what it seems to mean. It does not mean measures intended to keep disease from developing. Western Medicine does not believe in that. It takes disease for granted. Within the framework of Western Medicine, preventive medicine means early detection of disease. It means more frequent visits to the doctor's office, it means more frequent medical check-ups. This way, if there is something wrong, the doctor will be able to detect it early and to nip it in the bud.

Trouble is that, no matter how frequent these check-ups, they do not build health. For, if there is really something wrong and the doctor actually finds it, he will merely do what he has been trained to do -- patch up health that has begun to break down. The only thing that can be said in its favor is that, if a breakdown is detected early, a smaller "patch" will do. But it remains patching up, no matter the terminology. The emphasis is still on correction, not on prevention. Correction however is expensive and of limited effectiveness. And preventive medicine interpreted this way actually means more, not less business for the medical establishment, without any real improvement in popular health.

Let us look at two specific health problems to see what "preventive" steps Western Medicine would take and how Naturopathy would deal with the problems -- high blood pressure and heart disease.

Western Medicine classifies high blood pressure as a disease whose cause is not known and for which there is no known cure. The best it can do is control it -- with drugs, of course. In keeping with Western Medicine's view of preventive medicine, early drug therapy is standard dogma. Three types of drugs are used, separately or in combination -- 1) diuretics, 2) drugs that relax peripheral blood vessels and thereby reduce resistance to blood flow, and 3) drugs that act on the sympathetic nervous system. Usually the initial drug -- the one with the fewest side effects --is a diuretic. Diuretics reduce the volume of blood in the cardiovascular system by promoting fluid excretion via the kidneys. Less blood in the system means lower blood pressure. It actually seems to work with most patients. But it does so only as long as the drug is used. ***When the drug is discontinued, the blood pressure shoots up again***. However prolonged use of a diuretic poses problems. For one, by promoting fluid excretion, a diuretic also increases the excretion of several minerals, particularly potassium and magnesium.

There is, moreover, the problem of "accommodation" -- the fact that in time the body gets used to a given dosis of a diuretic and a stronger dosis is needed to produce the intended effect. This happens again and again, and the dosis must be progressively increased. But with higher doses, side effects are aggravated. Here are some of the side effects associated with prolonged use of diuretics: gastric pains, diarrhea, nausea, constipation; sexual impotence, disturbances in the menstrual cycle; skin problems; weight loss. For many patients, diuretic therapy becomes a terrible frying-pan-or-fire dilemma: continuing the drug means the continued risk of side effects; discontinuing the therapy means a return of the dreaded high blood pressure.

The naturopath does not regard high blood pressure as a disease of unknown cause nor yet as one for which there is no cure. In most cases the real cause of high blood pressure is very simply a faulty lifestyle; the remedy is to replace that lifestyle with one that is conducive to good health. The rest will take care of itself.

In general terms, a lifestyle conducive to good health means practicing the seven strategies discussed below. Particular emphasis would have to be placed on a wholesome diet, aerobic exercise, adequate rest, a low salt intake, weight reduction where necessary, the elimination of eliminable stresses and the consumption of natural remedies such as garlic, cayenne and celery. In 19 out of 20 cases, this approach would take care of the problem. And not only would there be no nasty side effects, there would be an all-round improvement of the patient's health.

Practicing the seven strategies of healthful living would be the most effective kind of preventive medicine for the heart too. He who practices them conscientiously can bid permanent farewell to the fear of a heart attack.

Western Medicine has more sophisticated ways of dealing with the problem -- all manner of medications; by-pass surgery (implanting healthy arteries in place of coronary arteries that have been clogged); angioplasty (inflating a small balloon that has been inserted in a clogged artery to stretch it); open heart surgery or even heart transplants. One British heart specialist made medical history a number of years ago by announcing that he had discovered a sure-fire way to prevent heart attacks -- one or two aspirins a day. Aspirin supposedly thins the blood to such an extent that no clots can form. No clots, no blocked arteries. No blocked arteries, no heart attacks. The British medical man was so taken by his discovery that he recommended the aspirin prophylaxis for every man above thirty and for every woman after menopause. "If," says the Britisher, "they take one or two aspirins every day of their lives, the risk of heart attacks becomes minimal."

Now, that is medicine gone mad. It takes heart attacks for granted. It suggests that our hearts cannot make it through the second half of life unless we consume some aspirin every day. I for one would rather have a healthy heart and healthy arteries than the doubtful protection of acetylsalicylic acid. For, even if the aspirin should protect me against a heart attack, the drug is not nearly as innocuous as the pharma-industry would have us believe. Among the possible side effects are gastrointestinal bleeding, nausea, vomiting, ringing of the ears, dizziness, hearing loss, liver damage, allergic skin reactions, asthma and drowsiness. But, even if the patient should escape all the side effects of the drug -- not likely with prolonged use! -- this sort of therapy does harm in that it prevents the patient from adapting a truly healthful lifestyle, with special emphasis on aerobic exercise. Surely that cannot be the intended meaning of preventive medicine -- that it should prevent the patient from becoming healthy.

      Western Medicine argues that it would be useless to ask patients to change their lifestyle because the majority of them would not listen anyway. How easy to believe what it is to one's advantage to believe! Western Medicine expends much effort and spends much money on selling its services -- immunization, semi-annual check-ups, blood pressure therapies, prophylactic hysterectomies (with prophylactic mastectomies in the offing), etc. If it invested half as much money and effort in campaigns to promote health, surely people would listen. An agency which has as much power over people's minds as Western Medicine, which can talk millions of women into permitting vital parts of their bodies to be cut away in (often unnecessary) hysterectomies and mastectomies -- could that same agency not get those same women to listen if it told them to exercise? If Western Medicine told people in clear language -- no pussy-footing, no obfuscation -- that they cannot hope to build health or to maintain it unless they correct their faulty lifestyle, surely many would listen. If doctors told prospective heart attack victims "You have a choice -- conventional patch-up procedures or real cure... real cure means exercise, a reasonable diet, adequate rest, etc.," many would listen.

      Not much chance, though, that Western Medicine will all of a sudden start to promote genuine health. Western Medicine *qua* big business cannot be expected to subordinate its own interests to those of society any more than big business in general. The only hope is for governments to step in. And here are a few things governments can or rather <u>must</u> do. They must change the status of the doctor, where this has not already been done, from that of a free-enterprise businessman to that of a salaried professional. A second thing governments must do is to put pressure on their respective medical establishments to switch from corrective to genuinely preventive medicine -- to teach their patients how to live so that eventually they won't get sick any more. It should be made mandatory for every doctor to have in his waiting room a pamphlet outlining the basic strategies of building health. Every patient should be given a copy of it to read. Those who cannot read should be made to listen to a taped version of it. And every patient should be told: "The ball is in your court. Play it. If you are not willing to do so, don't come back. Don't waste your doctor's time by getting sick. Getting sick is very unwise from a personal point of view. Getting sick is unethical in the light of the needs of society. Getting sick is very unpatriotic in the light of your country's needs."

And governments must introduce some accountability into medi-business. Virtually every line of non-medical business offers some sort of warranty for goods sold or services rendered. Medi-business does not. The doctor who would refuse to pay the mechanic if the car he was contracted to fix did not work expects, and gets, payment for a service that does not do what it is supposed to do, nay expects payment for a medical service that leaves the patient worse off than before or in extreme cases even medicates him to death.

Eventually, all these things and more will have to happen. Until they do, however, consider giving Naturopathic Medicine a try. There, virtually all those things have already happened. Perhaps we should go back to the system of health care practiced in ancient China, where a doctor received regular fees from his patients as long as they remained healthy. When a patient fell ill, he stopped paying and did not resume paying until his health was restored. Such a system offers financial rewards for health, not for disease. The doctor with the greatest number of healthy patients gets the biggest rewards. In Western Medicine it is the other way around. The greater the number of sick patients, the bigger the financial reward.

IV

SEVEN STRATEGIES OF WHOLESOME LIVING

Living so that eventually one won't need drugs or doctors means, generally speaking, creating for one's body an environment that is in keeping with the laws of its nature. More specifically it means practicing the following basic strategies of wholesome living:

1. sound nutrition
2. adequate exercise
3. adequate rest
4. relaxation
5. cleanliness
6. an occasional fast
7. a positive outlook

These are the seven strategies of wholesome living which represent the bedrock of Naturopathic Medicine. If you practice them reasonably conscientiously, you will stay healthy if you are healthy; if you are not, these same strategies will restore your health. It is as simple as that. Don't let any salesman of drugs or any medical man more interested in his stipend than in your health tell you otherwise.

> Then God said, "I give you every seed-bearing plant on the face of the earth and every tree that

has fruit with seed in it. They will be yours for food and healing." (GENESIS 1:29)

Strategy 1: sound nutrition Proper nutrition is probably the most important one of these strategies. You may think food is food. You may think that there is no significant difference other than taste between natural food and highly processed and refined food. But your body won't be fooled. If you prefer easy convenience foods to foods you have to prepare yourself -- corn flakes instead of hot whole-grain cereal for breakfast, a hamburger and chips or a roll made of white flour instead of steamed fish on brown rice and a raw vegetable salad for lunch, ice-cream instead of home-made yogurt and fruit for a late-afternoon snack -- you pay a doubly steep price: immediately, in terms of dollars, Riyals or Naira, for the food processor makes you pay for his labor of denaturing your food; and later, in terms of lost health.

It is amazing how little the majority of people even in developed countries know about nutrition. Perhaps I should have said it is amazing how much people know about nutrition that is wrong and harmful thanks to the corporate food processor's high pressure advertising. Take that very common piece of nutritional misinformation that we need sugar for energy. Here the advertising magician in the pay of the sugar lobby deliberately packs two terms into one as though they were one and the same thing -- *sugar* and *blood sugar* -- in order to confuse and to mislead. For, while it is true that the level of one's energy rises and falls with the concentration of glucose (blood sugar) in one's blood, it is equally true that putting refined white sugar into one's stomach is a quick and sure way of unbalancing one's sugar metabolism; and it makes no difference whether the sugar comes from the sugar bowl, from ice-cream, from pastry or from a soft drink.

Similar nutritional misinformation is put abroad by the makers of other highly processed and/or refined foods. A great many supermarket shoppers believe that white bread is good food because they are told that it has been enriched with vitamins, or that corn flakes are a good source of protein. In North America, where corn flakes used to be advertised as a good protein food, the makers of corn flakes had to change their tune owing to a court injunction. So they changed an outright lie to a half-lie by adding IF TAKEN WITH MILK to the original statement. But that had not affected the Nigerian scene by the time I left there, the spring of 1987. <u>Nestle's Golden Morn</u> still came in boxes that had HIGH PROTEIN printed on them in bold letters. How long, I wonder, before people will believe that synthetic food is better than real food, that imitation egg is better than real egg...?

If you pick up a cookbook, a book on nutrition or a textbook of Home Economics and you find it does not outlaw such denatured foods as white flour, white sugar, semovita, etc., put that book down. It is not for you. Cookbooks that tempt with irresistible compositions of junk food -- sweet cakes, cookies, gooey deserts, ice-cream, etc., all of them made of ingredients that supply virtually nothing but empty calories and undesirable additives -- put those books down. Look for books that stress the importance of whole foods, that teach you how to make delicious compositions of natural foods. Nutrition experts --

dieticians, teachers of Home Economics, teachers of Nutrition -- spend years studying the ins and outs of nutrition and yet they miss the most important consideration of all -- that one should, as much as possible, eat one's food whole, unrefined and unprocessed. All other considerations are secondary, even the question what to eat. For, if all, or at least most, of one's food is whole, unrefined and unprocessed, chances are that one gets all the nutrients one needs. In animal experiments, those fed a diet of whole grain and water remain healthy almost indefinitely while those fed on white flour or semovita and water soon sicken and die.

Therefore eat all your food in as natural a state as possible. And eat the *whole* food -- eat the whole orange rather than just drinking the juice of it; eat peanuts with their skins; eat tomatoes rather than drinking tomato juice; when possible, use tomatoes in your cooking, not tomato paste; eat potatoes, not potato chips ; eat the whole corn (maize) rather than corn flakes. If you live in a developing country, don't be ashamed to eat locally grown millet. Let others think you old-fashioned for eating old-fashioned food from the farm instead of packaged food from the supermarket. If you stick to your food-from-the farm resolution, you are going to reap big benefits of good health; they -- those who eat the highly processed and refined foods -- are setting their course for disease.

Every day try to eat raw some food that can be eaten raw -- some fruit, a tomato or two, a few carrots, lettuce, a cucumber. All processing of food, even cooking, destroys some nutrients. Raw food is unprocessed food and therefore has its nutrients intact.

If you cook your food, some vitamins and virtually all minerals survive but all enzymes are killed. And enzymes make all the difference.

I eat almost all my food raw, even meat. Of course I don't take a piece of raw meat and take bites of it like a carnivorous animal. I cure it, much as the meat that goes into Italian or Hungarian salami is cured, then cut it up fine and eat it with my salad of home-sprouted seeds. Delicious.

Avoid such non-foods as sugar, white-flour pastry, white rice, most of the finger foods put before you at parties, soft drinks, etc. Not only do they not contribute any nutrients to the body's ecology, they actually rob the body of nutrients. Everything we eat or drink has to be processed in the body. But, for this processing the body needs certain vitamins and minerals. Whole foods come well-provisioned with vitamins and minerals; in fact, they carry more of them than is needed for their own processing, and what is left over after they have been processed is credited to the body's nutritional bank account. Now the non-foods listed above not only do not supply the vitamins, enzymes or minerals required to process them: to process them, the body must dip into its own reserves of nutrients. Thus these offending substances -- they don't deserve to be called food or drink -- ***rob*** the body of vital nutrients instead of supplying them. Every cup of coffee costs in terms of the B-vitamins; sugar robs the body of B-vitamins and of certain minerals such as calcium, magnesium and potassium. You make matters worse if you take your coffee with sugar. If you do so, you send two nutritional thieves to prey on your body at the same time. A coke is much like a strong cup of coffee with lots of sugar.

But sugar, soft drinks -- in fact, all highly refined foods -- harm you in yet another way: they crowd out good food that would supply essential nutrients. When you are hungry, you should eat foods that supply what your body needs of building materials and nutrients. Natural foods like whole grain products, vegetables, fruit, etc. do that. The non-foods discussed above don't. With the calories they supply, they take your appetite away for the good foods, which would bring to your body what it needs of nutrients..

Go easy on the salt shaker. A high salt intake is the root of several ills, chief among them high blood pressure.

Don't eat several different foods at the same sitting. Different foods require different digestive juices. Carbohydrate foods require an alkaline environment while protein foods require an acid environment for optimal digestion. But the stomach cannot be alkaline and acid at the same time; in fact, these two substances neutralize each other. So, if you eat protein foods with starchy foods -- steak and potatoes, for instance -- digestion is either inhibited or arrested altogether. Instead of digesting, the mixture of foods in the stomach starts to decompose and to ferment. In the process gases are produced, which may leave you feeling bloated and bilious. Small quantities of alcohol may be produced, which can leave you feeling drowsy and out of sorts. Therefore, as much as possible, do not eat protein foods and carbohydrates at the same time. If you must have the steak and the potatoes, eat the former at noon and the latter in the evening. You may eat vegetables with either proteins or carbohydrates, but do not eat fruit and vegetables at the same time. Fruit, in fact, is best eaten by itself, on an empty stomach or between meals. Absolutely the worst thing you can do is to have a sweet dessert right after a protein-rich meal If you must have something sweet – this, by the way, applies to fruit too – have it between meals, not right after a meal.

Do not drink with your meals. Drink up to half an hour before a meal and not again till half an hour to an hour afterwards. When you eat, your saliva glands secrete saliva, which gets mixed with the food as your teeth grind it into pulp. This way the food becomes soft and slippery and it can be swallowed easily. But saliva serves a second purpose, probably more important than the first one. There are enzymes in saliva which are important for the digestion of food. If they are properly mixed with the food in the mouth, digestive processes are initiated even before the food reaches the stomach. But if you drink while you eat, your saliva glands get lazy. No need for them to exert themselves producing saliva. Lots of fluid coming in to make the food soft and moist for easy swallowing. But, no saliva, no predigesting of the food on its way to the stomach. An important part of the digestive process is aborted.

There is a second reason why you should not drink with your meals. A healthy stomach contains a delicately balanced mixture of digestive juices, all of them present in the right concentration. If you drink, that delicate balance is disturbed. The mixture gets diluted, the concentration of its various components is lowered. As a result, food cannot be effectively digested -- not until the natural concentration of the digestive juices is restored. Meanwhile the food in the stomach begins to deteriorate: it ferments, it starts to rot. In the process some nutrients are destroyed. Flatulence is a frequent side effect -- trapped gas rumbling up and down the intestines accompanied by frequent breaking of wind. Indigestion is another possible side effect.

After these general comments, here are some specific suggestions as to what to eat for people who would like to eat themselves into good health. Let us begin with <u>seeds and cereals.</u> Nature packs a lot of nutritional punch into seeds to ensure germination. Seeds include not only things which are actually called "seeds" such as sesame seeds, sunflower seeds and cotton seeds; they also include peas and beans, nuts and peanuts, wheat and millet and sorghum and any other food cereal you can think of.

Unrefined "seeds" are excellent breakfast cereals. Who needs cornflakes when he can have a bowl of cracked wheat topped with a mashed ripe banana? You can buy your cracked whole wheat at just about any grocery store. Take a portion of this cracked wheat, add a pinch of salt and soak it overnight. It will take very little cooking in the morning -- no more than ten minutes over a low flame. When it has cooled a bit, spread the mashed banana over it and dig in. It is delicious and marvelously nutritious.

Every now and then switch to a different grain such as millet or sorghum for a few days. Though the three kinds of grain are roughly comparable in their nutritional composition, each of them has its strengths and weaknesses. By switching, you can get the strength of one to compensate for the weakness of the other. For a change -- culinary and nutritional -- mix the three grains in equal parts. Should you not find cracked sorghum or millet in your neighborhood stores, use them whole. Wash the whole grains and soak them overnight. The next day, boil them as you would boil rice.

Another delicious and wholesome way of getting one's daily ration of "seeds" is whole-wheat bread. But keep what you don't eat immediately refrigerated because whole-wheat bread spoils rather quickly if it is not refrigerated. Want to know why whole-wheat bread does not keep as well as white bread? The answer is simple: spoilage bacteria love whole-wheat bread because it is chock-full of nutrients; they don't like white bread nearly as much because it has been robbed of most of its nutritional goodness. Unlike human beings, spoilage bacteria, in their instinctive wisdom, know what's good for them.

If you can't find, or want to save yourself the trouble of hunting for, genuine whole-wheat bread, why don't you bake your own? Using my quick-and-easy recipe a few pages down, you won't mind baking your own. Baking your own has several advantages: you can have your bread oven-fresh every day; you can, after a little experimenting, bake the kind of bread that appeals to you both in texture and flavor; and your bread will be guaranteed free of undesirable additives.

Why this insistence on whole-wheat bread? Reference has been made to animal experiments which demonstrated that a diet of whole wheat and water is sufficient to keep animals healthy almost indefinitely, while a diet of water and any of the refined-wheat products soon makes them sick and eventually kills them. Now, if human beings were subjected to the same conditions, we would see the same results: those on whole wheat would do well, while those on white bread would sicken and eventually die. But human beings do not normally live on refined-wheat products alone. They have other foods in their diets which make up for the deficiency. That's why they can go on eating those denatured foods for a long time without becoming aware how, every time they do eat white bread or pastry, they short-change themselves nutritionally.

In developed countries it is generally true that the poorer the people, the bigger the part played by refined wheat products in their total food consumption. Accordingly the damage done among them is greater -- damage in terms of lower resistance to disease; damage in terms of reduced efficiency of functioning on the physical, the emotional and mental levels; damage in terms of premature aging and reduced life expectancy.

In developing countries, the refined-wheat products have something of the status-symbol glow about them. Everybody wants them, though not everybody can afford them. Ironically people have to reach a certain socio-economic level before they can afford to inflict on themselves the hygienic insult of the refined-wheat products, while the poorest of the poor, who cannot afford them, have to settle for the despised but wholesome millet or unpolished rice.

Ironic too that those refined-wheat products should have come to play so big a part in developing countries, where people can least afford them -- can't afford them from an economic point of view, can't afford them from a nutritional point of view. Where the specter of hunger is the daily companion of millions of people, one cannot afford to throw away 20 per cent of the available wheat. Yet 20 per cent is roughly what's lost in the milling. Twenty per cent of a million tons would be 200,000 tons.

The figures don't tell the whole story. The twenty per cent refers only to the volume of the portion lost in milling. It says nothing about the fact that the lost portion contains most of the nutritional goodness of the wheat.

The wheat berry consists of three separable parts -- the outer covering or the bran, the germ, and the carbohydrate core. The first two contain most of the nutritional goodness, but they are discarded; the carbohydrate core, the part that is turned into human food, consists of little more than naked calories.

Wheat germ is a veritable gold mine of good nutrition. It contains protein of a high quality. The fat it contains is good for the heart and blood vessels. It is, besides, our best dietary source of Vitamin E, a vitamin so important in human nutrition that whole books have been written about it. Wheat germ rivals liver and the nutritional yeasts as one of the best sources of virtually all the known B-vitamins. Wheat germ finally contains the bulk of the minerals found in whole wheat, among them iron, manganese, magnesium, selenium and copper.

There is something else in wheat germ, something researchers have termed "anti-stress factors." Though these factors have not been positively identified, their existence has been amply demonstrated in animal experiments. They protect against a variety of stresses. If, for instance, rats are fed certain harmful substances in doses that could be counted on to do harm -- strychnine, sulfanilamide, silbesterol, cortisone, aspirin and other drugs -- those animals which are given foods containing the stress factors are surprisingly immune to the noxious substances. Anti-stress factors have been shown to exist in liver and some of the nutritional yeasts. The forte of the anti-stress factors contained in wheat germ seems to be their ability to increase resistance to bacterial infections. There is evidence that the anti-stress factors increase resistance to the harmful effects of radiation, both radioactive and X-ray.

    Pages could be written about the health benefits of wheat bran. On one hand, it is itself a good source of the B-vitamins. It supplies significant quantities of B1, B2, B3, Biotin, Choline, Pantothenic acid and Folic acid. It also supplies significant quantities of various minerals. But the real importance of bran lies in the contribution it makes to health as fiber; it is, in fact, our best dietary source of fiber.

    Fiber is the undigested part of carbohydrates. Its main role is to provide bulk for the feces. On diets low in fiber, feces become hard. Constipation results. And constipation is the root of many ills, among them diverticulosis and diverticulitis, hemorrhoids, varicose veins and probably arthritis. Besides, fiber acts as a carrier of many substances through the intestinal tract, substances both good and bad. Heavy metals are among the bad substances. By binding them, fiber decreases their chances of harming the intestine or being absorbed into the blood stream.

A diet rich in fiber is probably good protection against cancer of the colon. Cancer of the colon is rare in areas where people live on fiber-rich diets, while the incidence of cancer of the colon is high in areas where people live on diets of refined foods that are poor in fiber. The evidence is only circumstantial. Still, I put my bets on fiber. If it does not help, at least it won't do any harm.

So, wheat germ and bran are the two parts of the wheat kernel that carry the nutritional punch. Yet they are discarded while the white part, which is hardly fit for human consumption, is turned into food for human beings. Why? It cannot be ignorance. The flour millers of the 19th century were probably convinced that they did humanity a service by producing a food that looked good, tasted good and kept well. They were ignorant of the nutritional implications of their work. Today ignorance can no longer be adduced as an excuse. The corporate flour millers know all there is to know about their business. They know that their milling turns an excellent food into something that does not deserve to be classed as food any longer. Yet they persist in their nutritional perversity.

They do so because there is big money in it. The syndicate of wheat growers, flour millers and makers of refined wheat products, chief among them white bread, represent a multi-billion dollar business that reaches into the most remote corners of our globe. And the financial success of the operation can be attributed largely to the very fact that the refined wheat products have little nutritional value. That's why even spoilage bacteria stay away from them. That's why they can be stored in warehouses almost indefinitely. That's why they can be shipped over long distances in unrefrigerated vehicles without risk of spoilage. Whole-wheat products, by contrast, spoil quickly. They must therefore be consumed quickly or refrigerated. Refrigerating them on a large scale would be expensive. Imagine all the fridge space one would need to refrigerate all the bread sold in a country like Nigeria!

The other cereals available in many of the developing countries -- millet, sorghum, maize -- are not readily made into bread. They lack gluten, the stuff that is responsible for the stickiness of wheat. A thick paste of wheat flour and water actually makes a good glue. It is this gluten that makes bread hold together; and, since millet, sorghum and maize don't have it, one cannot readily make bread from them.

However, in terms of their nutritional value, those other cereals compare favorably with wheat. Provided they are consumed whole, nothing taken away, they are excellent foods. The following table, taken from the US Agriculture Handbook of Foods, shows how similar sorghum is to wheat in its nutritional make-up:

Food	Calories	Protein	Fat	Carbohydrates	Fiber
Wheat	330	14	2.2	69	2.3
Sorghum	332	11	3.0	73	2.3

During World War II, the government of Denmark passed a law that prohibited the refining of wheat. The objective of the measure was to make the wheat supply go further by saving for human consumption the 20 % or so of the grain removed in the milling process. After the war, when scientists set out to study the effect of the war measure on popular health, they came to the conclusion that the shift to whole wheat had resulted in a significant reduction of the general death rate. It took another decade before the bio-science community was ready to venture an explanation for the phenomenon -- that it was the retention for human nutrition of all the B-vitamins and of Vitamin E, of various minerals and of the dietary fiber contained in the wheat germ and the bran that had made the difference.

At this point I would like to appeal to governments the world over to consider following the example Denmark set under the pressure of wartime necessity -- to forbid the general refining of wheat. It could be done. Existing flour mills can produce whole-wheat flour as well as white flour. And the savings would be incalculable -- savings in terms of volume, savings in terms of improved general health.

Let me conclude this discussion of seeds and cereals by giving you my recipe for a delicious home-made whole-wheat bread. It is simplicity itself. I had long shied away from baking my own whole-wheat bread because all the recipes I had ever come across seemed too much trouble. But in my African setting, it became a case of do or die. When I first got there, in 1980, there was no whole-wheat bread to be had anywhere. The local white bread was even worse -- if that's possible -- than the North American white toast bread. To the denatured white flour, the makers of the local bread added the hygienic insult of lots of sugar, presumably to make the bread taste better and to "give the consumer energy." The result was a nutritional disaster. After a closer look at it, I decided that I would rather live without bread than eat that. And I did live without bread for some time. Eventually I gave in. I bought wheat at the market, had it ground into coarse whole-wheat flour at a local put-put mill and started to experiment. In time I developed a recipe that is both simple and effective. Here it is.

Throw into a bowl or basin

> 2 1/2 cups of whole-wheat flour
> 1/2 t of salt
> 3/4 T of baking powder
> some powdered milk.

Mix the dry ingredients well. Then add a little cooking oil -- 3 to 5 tablespoons. Work the oil into the flour with a spoon or with your hands. Make sure you leave no oil-soaked lumps of flour. Then add water -- about 1 1/2 cups of it. Work the water in with a sturdy spoon. When you are done, you should have a dough that is a little too wet to be worked by hand but not runny. No kneading is necessary. Experiment with a little more and a little less fluid. You will see that, all else being equal, a little more fluid will give you a somewhat fluffier bread; a little less fluid will give you a bread that is more compact. Both the fluffier and the more compact varieties, and anything that is in-between, are deliciously eatable.

Instead of the water, you may use fruit that has been liquefied in a blender or mashed or grated. I have used ripe bananas, papaya, mango, pineapple and peaches. Again, experiment. Use part water and part liquefied fruit. The addition of fruit changes both the texture and the flavor of your bread. The result is a kind of bread that is ideal for breakfast. It is nice as a snack in the afternoon, to be taken with a cup of herbal tea.

The baking of it? Well, you have a choice of two approaches. (1) You throw little lumps of the dough on a greased cookie sheet, flatten them so that they end up being about 1 1/2 inches thick. Then bake them in the oven.

(2) If you have no oven, you can "bake" your bread in an oven substitute -- a heavy, cast-iron frying pan. Grease the pan lightly. Then proceed as with the lumps on the cookie sheet. Cover and bake over very low heat. If you have a gas stove, the very lowest flame is just right. Bake for about 15 minutes on one side; then turn the "lumps" over and bake for another ten minutes on the other side....

<u>Vegetables</u> are generally low in calories and rich in essential nutrients –- vitamins, minerals, fiber. They are besides a source of various enzymes, substances which play a vital role in many digestive processes.

If at all possible, you should eat some vegetables every day. And you should eat as many of them as possible raw. Cooking destroys some of the nutrients. Vegetables lose some of their nutrients during prolonged storage. Only raw vegetables fresh from the garden contain their full complement of nutrients.

Now, while most vegetables are best eaten raw, some of them such as carrots, squash and turnips yield more of their nutritional goodness if either cooked or juiced. The cellulose of their cell walls is so tough that the human digestive system cannot fully break them down. Cooking helps. But you should not overcook them, and you should not throw out the water used to cook the vegetables.

Sometimes I juice my carrots. Juicing them extracts all the nutritional goodness out of the tough fiber without destroying the enzymes. And freshly extracted carrot juice is absolutely delicious. But you need a juicer for that. You can't juice carrots in a blender.

The most palatable way of eating raw vegetables is a salad. Here is a suggestion for a delicious raw salad:

      1/2 head of lettuce
      1 medium onion

    1 or two tomatoes
    1 or 2 peppers, green or red, <u>chopped</u>
    1 or 2 small cucumbers
    1 or 2 carrots, <u>grated</u>

    2 T of unpasteurised vinegar
    2 T of extra-virgin olive oil
    2 T of soy sauce
    a sprinkle of black or red pepper
    1 T of roasted sesame seeds.

If you crumble one or two hard-boiled eggs into this salad, you have a meal. I often have this kind of salad for breakfast.

    Juicing vegetables is perhaps even better than eating them in a salad. My favorites are carrot juice and celery juice, on one hand because they are easy to juice and on the other hand because they are veritable gold mines of nutritional benefits. Do a web search for the benefits of either and you'll be surprised by what you will discover. Among other things you will learn that Celery juice contains several ingredients that are credited with fighting cancer.

    It is good policy to eat whatever happens to be in season and therefore cheapest. In my African setting, vegetables became scarce and expensive during the latter half of the long dry season and the first couple of months of the rainy season. In the bigger cities, some vegetables could be found, but they were expensive and, because they came from far away, they were not all too fresh. Friends of mine who worked in the "bush" simply could not get vegetables at all. However, city or bush, there was a way we could get fresh vegetables for our dinner table even then, cheaply and reliably -- sprouted seeds. Sprouted seeds recommend themselves anywhere as a highly nutritious food; in the Sahel Zone they were invaluable.

    You can sprout almost any edible seeds. Beans, cereal grains such as wheat, sorghum, corn, sesame seeds, peanuts -- they all work. I have found mung beans and lentils the most rewarding sprouters Most Saudi supermarkets carry them. Four tablespoons of dry seeds turn into a quart-bowl of crisp "vegetables" when sprouted.

Here is the lazy man's way of sprouting seeds. Get yourself a sieve no less than six inches in diameter. Perhaps get two -- a colander for the bigger seeds such as lentils, beans, peanuts and sorghum, and a fine-mesh one for the smaller seeds like alfalfa and sesame seeds. Cover the bottom of the sieve with seeds. Wash them thoroughly and remove foreign objects. Then set the sieve with the seeds in a basin -- the sink will do -- containing enough water to cover the seeds. Let them soak overnight. In the morning, lift the sieve out of the water. Rinse the seeds thoroughly by running clean cold water over them. Then cover the sieve with a plate and put it in a cool place. If you are in the tropics, an air-conditioned room is best; for, if they get too warm, they go bad easily unless you rinse them very frequently. Here, in my Nova Scotia mid-latitude setting, I simply keep them in the sink.

Now all you have to do for the next three or four days is to rinse the seeds frequently, say at least six times a day. I leave mine in a place where I cannot possibly overlook and so forget to rinse them. If I put them out of sight, I inevitably forget to rinse them and they spoil. Frequent rinsing assures that the sprouts stay crisp and fresh.

Before the end of the second day, tiny sprouts should appear. After three to four days, when the sprouts have reached a length of about an inch, they are ready to eat.

You can eat the sprouts by themselves, add them to salads or put them into stews. I have had many a salad consisting of nothing but sprouts, olive oil and soy sauce. If you want to put your sprouts in a stew, cook the stew first. When it is almost done, add the sprouts and set it to simmer for a few more minutes. Much cooking would destroy too much of their nutritional goodness.

Sprouts are the equivalent of the best of fresh vegetables. There is convincing evidence that the vitamin content of seeds, which is exceptionally high to begin with, increases manifold in sprouting. Sprouts are such a powerhouse of good nutrition that, if one had to live on them exclusively, one could survive and stay healthy for a long time.

Much of what has been said of vegetables is true of <u>fruit</u> -- that they are rich in vitamins, minerals and enzymes, that they are a good source of dietary fiber. As much as reasonably possible, they should be eaten WHOLE -- skin and pulp and seeds and all. I said "as much as reasonably possible." You don't want to eat the skin of a banana or of a pineapple. However there is no need to peel a guava, a mango or an apple. As for oranges, don't just juice them. Peel them, by all means, but eat the whole fruit that comes out of the peel. And dig some of the white lining out of the peel. It is the richest source available of the bioflavonoids, which are part of the Vitamin C complex.

In my African setting, I grew some fruit of my own. Papaya was my favorite. A papaya tree grows to fruit-bearing maturity in less than a year. I planted my first papaya seedlings on Dec. 20, 1980. About nine months later, they were more than 12 feet tall and heavy with fruit. By the beginning of December 1981 I had eaten the first of my own papayas. And the two trees kept supplying me with fruit for the next four months.

Nor is growing your own fruit just a matter of economy. It enables you to pick the fruit at its best. There is no comparison between a tree-ripened papaya and one which, picked green, ripens in a fruit vendor's stall. I planted a guava and a mango tree though I knew full well that I would not be there by the time they'd bear fruit. I was happy to think that someone else would get to enjoy their fruit.

When we talk of protein foods most people think of meat, eggs and dairy products. In fact, many people believe that to fill one's protein needs, one must have meat and milk or eggs every day. Not so. If one's diet consists largely of unrefined foods of plant origin, one does not need to worry whether one gets enough protein. Practically all unrefined plant foods contain some protein; some of them -- beans, peanuts, nuts and other seeds – are good sources of protein. If you live on a varied diet of unrefined plant foods, you get all you need of protein. It is the people whose diet consists largely of refined foods -- foods composed of white flour, white sugar and other junk -- that need to worry about their protein intake.

And you can safely ignore the outworn myth that your body can make use of the protein you ingest *qua* protein only if you obtain all the essential amino acids at the same meal. True, your body may not be able to produce any of these so-called essential amino acids, but the liver can store the ones that come in till the missing ones arrive and then proceed to synthesize complete proteins. Not getting all the essential amino acids would be a problem only if an imbalance persisted for a long time -- if, for instance, your only source of protein were gelatin.

At this point, a word or two about vegetarianism may be in order. There are lots of vegetarians in the world, people who don't eat meat, and some of them are among the healthiest people we know. In Chapter I, I talked about the Hunza as a group of people who contrive to be so healthy that they don't need drugs or doctors. They can also serve as an illustration of people who contrive to be enviably healthy on a vegetarian diet. A long-term study by the German Cancer Research Center in Heidelberg, which followed nearly 2000 vegetarians over a period of eleven years, came to the conclusion that vegetarians not only enjoy better than average health but also have a greater life expectancy.

People are vegetarians for various reasons. Some are vegetarians for ideological reasons. They regard life as something too sacred to be destroyed merely to satisfy man's wanton appetites and to guaranty profits for the cattle breeders and the meat-processors. Millions of Indians subscribe to this philosophy.

In some parts of the world, people are vegetarians out of necessity. Where there is little arable land, people cannot afford to "grow" meat. The following model demonstrates why.

A given amount of grain, sufficient to feed 100 people, feeds 30 people if converted to beef and milk, feeds 12 people if converted to chicken and eggs, feeds 8 people if converted to pork.

The Hunza are vegetarians out of necessity. Hemmed in by the Himalayan Mountains, they have relatively little arable land. They can therefore not afford to convert their crops into meat. For them, meat is a luxury, which they permit themselves only on special occasions.

I believe that eventually the whole human race will have to adopt a diet much like that of the Hunza, with meat as an occasional treat rather than as a major source of food. In a world where hundreds of millions of people go to bed hungry day after day, where in fact millions of people starve to death every year, the kind of super-carnivorous lifestyle that is typical of the developed countries is indefensible. It is both wasteful and immoral. There would be more than enough to eat for everybody if the plant food which the West converts into meat were used directly to feed the hungry. In the West, "growing" meat is in fact one of several ways of getting rid of an embarrassing surplus of food.

There are, finally, people who adopt a vegetarian diet because they believe that it is more wholesome than a carnivorous diet. I call them the functional vegetarians. I am one of them myself. I lived on a purely vegetarian diet for ten years of my life and I have never felt better than I did then. If I have drifted back into eating meat it is because the woman who became my wife some 25 years ago would have refused to marry me if I had not compromised. We did eat meat, but we ate very little of it. For us meat served as a condiment rather than as a major source of food. A good many people in Africa follow a similar dietary approach, but they do so out of necessity, not by choice: they simply cannot afford to buy meat in big quantities. On my own now, I still eat a little meat but I cure it and eat it raw.

Though I privately believe that a vegetarian diet is more conducive to good health than a diet heavy on meat, it is not my intention to make a formal pronouncement here. I merely wish to reassure the reader that there is nothing wrong with a meatless diet provided that it is a balanced diet of unrefined plant foods.

Some time ago an anti-vegetarian friend of mine sent me a paper clipping about a New York couple that was admitted to hospital with symptoms of severe malnutrition. In spite of the best medical care, the wife died. The husband survived, but it took him weeks fully to recover.

The two, the clipping explained, had been living on a pure vegetarian diet of nothing but polished rice and water for several months in the belief that they would progress spiritually on such a diet. My friend, knowing that I was a vegetarian at the time, meant the clipping to serve as a warning to me. I wrote back: "Living on nothing but polished rice is not vegetarianism: it is nutritional idiocy."

After this digression on vegetarianism, back to the protein foods. Meat, eggs, dairy products -- these are the protein foods *par excellence*. But they tend to be expensive in developing countries. While I was in Nigeria, a day's wages of an unskilled laborer bought about 2 dozen eggs; at the time, a Canadian on minimum wage could buy some 15 dozen eggs for a day's wages.

If these protein foods were – and still are – very expensive in northern Nigeria, they were and are even more so in less developed parts of Africa. In many places they are either not available or so expensive that the common man cannot afford them.

Nevertheless, in the light of what I have said about vegetarianism, the poor in developing countries need not despair. They may be angry at not being given a chance to enjoy these luxury foods, but they need not despair of achieving good health without them. One can indeed be healthy without them. Lots of people the world over abstain from these foods voluntarily because they believe that a diet of plant foods is more conducive to good health than one containing significant quantities of meat.

All considered, eggs are the best of the protein foods. Eat three to four eggs a week if you can afford them. If you like eggs and would like to eat more of them, by all means do. \

Don't let the cholesterol scare deter you from eating eggs. True, the yolk of the egg contains much cholesterol, but it also supplies lecithin, a substance needed to keep cholesterol "honest." Moreover, what we get of cholesterol from our food has little effect on our blood cholesterol levels. Cholesterol is a vital substance, something the liver knows very well; for it produces most of it. We can abstain from foods containing cholesterol altogether and end up with what the makers of the highly profitable statins – cholesterol-lowering drugs – class as high cholesterol levels. There are a good many studies which demonstrate that people with high cholesterol live longer. I, for one, am not in the least worried about my cholesterol.

A word or two about how to eat your eggs. Don't fry them. All fried foods are difficult to digest, and some researchers suspect them of being carcinogenic, especially if fried in vegetable oil. Boil your eggs, poach them, or – if you can -- eat them raw. I have one or two raw eggs every day. I bang them into a mug, beat them with a fork, add a little salt and beat them some more and then drink them, washing my fat-soluble vitamins down with them. A raw egg is the perfect food. It contains all the nutrients and building materials to create a new chick. Don't let fear of catching all sorts of germs keep you from having your egg(s) raw. I don't seem to have caught any in years and years of eating my eggs raw.

What I just said about frying eggs applies to meat: don't fry meat; if you cannot live without fried meat, at least do not consume fried meat regularly. The best way to cook meat is to boil it, as a great many Africans do anyway in the preparation of their many varieties of delicious meat-plus-vegetable stews. It is all right to grill or to roast meat every now and then.

Some kinds of meat are preferable to others. Organ meats (liver, heart, kidney, etc.) are preferable to muscle meats; fish and fowl are preferable to sheep and goat, which in turn are preferable to beef and pork.

Go easy on canned meat. Most varieties of canned meat contain undesirable additives, sugar among them.

And keep in mind that you should eat meat in moderation. Arguments pro or con vegetarianism aside, most nutrition experts agree that excessive meat consumption is not good in the long run. If you find a nutrition book that extols meat eating, have a second look. It is probably an American book. Lots of American nutrition books echo the pro-meat propaganda of the American beef-growers' lobby. As long as your diet is basically what it should be -- a balanced diet of natural foods -- the less meat you eat, the better.

In most of the poorer societies of the world, meat is a status symbol. The rich, who can afford to eat meat, eat it ostentatiously. And they consume big quantities of it. The poor have to content themselves with lowly cereals and vegetables, with perhaps a little meat for flavoring. The irony of it is that the ostentatious consumers of meat, while they may be able to afford the purchase price of meat, pay a price they can ill afford to pay -- impaired health; to wit, gout, early arthritis, early atherosclerosis, things which the meatless poor are relatively immune to. In medieval Europe, the feudal lords sat down to banquets of mainly meat and liquor. Foods of plant origin were beneath their dignity. Plant foods were for the serfs. But, irony of ironies, the grand mass of serfs were by and large lean and healthy, while their masters howled with the pain of gout before they were out of their thirties.

There remain the <u>dairy products</u> -- milk, yogurt and cheese. Like most foods, milk is best if consumed in as natural a state as possible. Fresh **raw** milk is best, provided it comes from healthy cows. In my African setting I had to compromise. If I could get fresh milk, I pasteurized it -- heated it to about 80° C and then let it cool again -- because I could not be sure that it came from certifiably healthy cows. When I could not get fresh milk -- which was most of the time -- I settled for the processed varieties of milk such as powdered or evaporated milk when they were available. I do not consider the fresh milk sold in our supermarkets good milk. Hands off condensed milk because of its high sugar content.

The nutritional value of milk is enhanced if it is made into <u>yogurt</u>. In fact, the processed varieties of milk -- evaporated milk, powdered milk -- which have lost some of their nutrients in the processing, can be "rehabilitated" to an extent if they are made into yogurt.

Yogurt has much to offer. It is a good source of high-quality protein, which moreover is more readily assimilated than the protein of plain milk because the yogurt bacteria have "predigested" it. Yogurt is besides a good source of calcium and it supplies significant amounts of the B-vitamins. The B-vitamins are manufactured by the same bacteria that convert milk into yogurt.

If yogurt had nothing further to offer, it would deserve a place on a list of valuable foods. But there is more to yogurt -- more than the nutrients it contains. You see, the very culture that transforms milk into yogurt is virtually identical with the intestinal flora of a healthy individual. That intestinal flora of friendly bacteria performs a number of important services for the host organism -- it assists in digestive processes, it manufactures significant quantities of various B-vitamins and Vitamin K, and it generally keeps the intestinal ecology in good condition. As long as the intestinal flora is intact, the individual is all but immune to intestinal disturbances. By the same token, good yogurt is good first aid for most common digestive-tract upsets. Yogurt insures that the intestinal flora remains intact or that it is restored if for whatever reason it has been compromised.

So the next time you are put on antibiotics, remember to put yourself on a supplementary yogurt regime. Your doctor, if he is trained in the American tradition of Western Medicine, is not likely to know. He is more likely to know if he had his training in one of the former socialist countries like Russia, Poland or Czechia. A doctor who prescribes antibiotics without telling his patient to take a few spoonfuls of good yogurt halfway through the time that separates the antibiotic intake is guilty of malpractice; morally, that is, if not legally. Big Pharma makes sure that he is legally protected.

Hands off the flavored varieties of yogurt sold in most supermarkets. They contain sugar and other undesirable additives. If you cannot get used to plain yogurt, create your own flavored varieties. Mashed bananas, strawberries or peaches combine deliciously with plain yogurt. And consider making your own yogurt. It is cheaper, it tastes better and it is better for you than the yogurts you buy in your supermarket. No need to buy a yogurt maker; you don't need one to make yogurt. Here is my own no-nonsense method of making yogurt, the result of much trial and error:

> Use any kind of milk –fresh milk, evaporated milk, cereal creme or powdered milk. If you want to use powdered milk, reconstitute it in lukewarm water in your blender. Add about two tablespoons of "starter" to a blender bowl. The starter, by the way, is merely plain yogurt. The first time you have to "import" a starter. Ideally you get a yogurt culture from a health food store. Failing that, look for a commercial yogurt that has not been pasteurized. A yogurt that has been ;asteurized won't work as a starter because sterilizing kills the bacterial culture that transforms milk into yogurt. But once you have your own yogurt, all you have to do is save an ounce or two from one batch to the next to use as a starter. Put the milk *cum* starter in a bowl, cover it and leave it in a warm place. While "incubating," its temperature should be somewhere between 80 F (27 C) and body temperature. If it is too cold, it won't "hatch"; if too hot, the starter dies and it won't "hatch" either. In either case you will end up with spoiled milk rather than yogurt. If conditions are right, it will make itself in 4 to 6 hours. Experiment with a few small batches first. When you have the hang of it, you can make big batches.

Yogurt can be eaten in a variety of ways: it can be eaten by itself; it can be eaten with fruit that has been cut up or mashed; it can be made into milk-shake-like drinks that are both highly nutritious and delicious. Yogurt is a food I would not want to live without.

<u>Cheese</u> is an excellent protein food too. It can readily take the place of meat in the nutritional balance. Cheese, moreover, has it over meat in that it doesn't contain uric acid, high levels of which can cause gout.

Unfortunately cheese tends to be rare and expensive in most developing countries. One can find it only in the biggest cities, and even there it is a now-and-then commodity.

Eat cheese if it is available in your area and if you can afford it. Cheese with a slice of fresh whole-wheat bread makes a delicious and nutritious snack. But don't despair if you cannot get cheese. Though it is one of our best foods, it is not essential to good health.

Special Foods. I have already dealt with some of the foods that I consider "special" from the point of view of good health -- yogurt, wheat germ, wheat bran and sprouted seeds. There are four more on my private list, whose praises I would like to sing -- liver, brewer's yeast, coconut oil and garlic.

I considered *liver* an important part of my stay-well program while I was in Africa. Before I went there, I had not eaten liver for many years, partly because I had lived on a vegetarian diet and partly because I felt I could do without liver. At home in Canada I routinely took high potency Vitamin A and B-complex supplements. Since I could not get those supplements in Africa, I settled for liver as a good alternative. For liver contains the whole range of the B-vitamins and it is at the same time one of the best sources of Vitamin A.

There are other reasons why I regard liver as one of the special foods. It represents a source of protein of the highest quality. It supplies moreover some of the anti-stress factors which I touched on briefly in connection with wheat germ. True, these anti-stress factors have not as yet been identified as such, but their existence has been demonstrated in animal experiments. It has been shown that liver increases resistance to stress and disease beyond what one would expect from the known nutrients it contains.

So, vegetarian or carnivore, you could do worse than eat a few ounces of liver now and then, perhaps as often as two or three times a week. All considered, liver is one of the best foods available to man.

I said above that liver is an excellent source both of the whole range of the B-vitamins and of Vitamin A. Liver is, in fact so rich in these vitamins that, if a deficiency were suspected, liver could be used therapeutically to correct it. Let me show you how true this is of liver qua source of Vitamin A. Suppose your doctor were to advise you to take a daily 10,000 IU (international units) of that vitamin for a month. That would mean a total of 300,000 IU. It would take .6 kg of liver to supply that amount since 1 kg of liver contains a whopping 500,000 IU. Now six-tenths of 1 kg for the whole month would work out to only 20 grams a day or 40 grams every second day, that is one or two slices about the size of the palm of your hand. And all that liver would cost you less than $ 6.-- at current prices.

While I was in Jeddah, Saudi Arabia, I inquired about Vitamin A at several pharmacies. None of them had anything more potent than 1,000 IU capsules. And they were SR 6.50 for 30. It would take ten a day of these capsules for a month -- a total of 300 -- to give you 300,000 IU. At SR 6.50 for 30, it would cost you SR 65.00. In the circumstances I would get my A from liver rather than from supplements. This way, I would pay much less for my A and I would get as a bonus all the nutritional goodness contained in liver in addition to Vitamin A.

Brewer's yeast is a by-product of beer brewing. It is, to be more precise, the yeast that causes the mash -- mixture of malt, hops and water -- to ferment. It is a close relative of the yeast used in bread baking. When the fermentation is over, the yeast is collected, dried and sold as a nutritional supplement.

Together with liver and wheat germ, brewer's yeast is one of the best dietary sources of the B-vitamins. It is, besides, a good source of high-quality protein. And, like liver and wheat germ, its two main rivals, brewer's yeast supplies the anti-stress factors. In various systems of North American and European folk medicine, brewer's yeast is held in very high esteem. Some people regard it as a panacea for all kinds of ills.

In North America and Europe, brewer's yeast is available in health food stores and in many pharmacies. I did not find it in Saudi Arabia, perhaps because of its association with beer, something that's illegal in that country. Brewer's yeast is not itself a vitamin; it is merely a food rich in some of the most important vitamins.

Coconut oil is truly one of the miracle foods. I take two or three tablespoons of it every day. If someone dear to me showed signs of dementia or Alzheimer's, coconut oil would be the first substance I'd reach for. I'd resort to coconut oil as an effective all-round "antibiotic" without side effects, one that could be trusted to combat the whole spectrum of disease-generating microbes, not just bacteria – yeast, fungi and viruses, even the HIV virus and the supposedly incurable herpes virus. Those battling overweight would do well to elect coconut oil as their ally. .

Fully to sing the praises of ***garlic*** would fill a book bigger than this one here. Let me but list summarily a few of its more striking properties. Garlic is an excellent regulator of blood pressure; it is one of the best expectorants and cough medicines available; it can be counted on to lower blood levels of cholesterol; it is an effective de-worming agent; and it has germicidal qualities comparable to those of an antibiotic. And all that without nasty side effects.

Two of these properties of garlic deserve a closer look -- the fact that it regulates blood pressure and its germicidal qualities.

In Saudi Arabia many people suffer from high blood pressure and many of them are on expensive antihypertensive drugs, often for years, which do very little good while they can have nasty side effects. Western Medicine admits readily that it has no cure for high blood pressure, that all it can do is control it. Now, in the chapter on preventive medicine I explained that there is indeed a cure for high blood pressure -- the only cure, and a sure cure at that -- the kind of lifestyle that would prevent the ill in the first place. But, if you are not willing to adopt such a lifestyle, there is still an alternative to drugs -- garlic. Two to three medium-sized cloves of garlic twice a day will do it. Don't expect it to work overnight. You'll have to keep at it for several weeks. But it will work. And it will work all the more effectively if you reduce your salt intake at the same time.

The garlic should be raw and fresh. If you cook garlic or if you keep it till it is old and yellow, it loses much of its healing power. Cut it up fine and eat it with your stews, with your salads, with any food really that is salty. You can take a few little pieces with each mouthful of food or you can actually stir the cut-up garlic right into the whole lot of food. You'll be surprised how good it tastes and how much it enhances the taste of most of your food. However, if you are one of the minority of people who dislike the taste of garlic so much that they cannot take it this way, here is how you can get enough garlic into you to be therapeutically effective without having to "eat" it: peel a few cloves... chop them finely... load the pieces on a spoon and put them in your mouth, as far back as possible... then wash them down, unchewed, with a little water, as you would wash down pills. If you can't do that either, take garlic pills.

Should you be worried about the smell of garlic on your breath, I have good news for you. If the garlic is fresh and raw, you will not smell after a few days, at most a week. When you first start to eat garlic, your body is not ready for it. It does not have the enzymes necessary for metabolizing it completely. But your body's biochemical ingenuity quickly remedies the deficiency -- the enzymes needed to metabolize garlic are produced and there is no more smell of garlic on your breath. Just one caution though --- to make sure your breath is wholly clean, brush your teeth after a "garlic" meal so as to remove garlic particles lodged there. If you take garlic pills, you don't even have to do that.

World-famous Dr. Albert Schweitzer was one of the first medical men in modern times to capitalize on the antibiotic qualities of garlic. When, during World War II, medical supplies from Europe failed him, he had to fall back on what was locally available. Garlic then became an important item in his pharmacy. Dr. Schweitzer made extensive use of it in the treatment of infections, especially infections of the gastro-intestinal tract. In more recent years, the Russians have done a great deal of research on the germicidal powers of garlic. In Russian medical practice, garlic takes its place side by side with established antibiotics.

Don't expect great things to happen in the West regarding the medical use of garlic. Medical research in the West is financed largely by the big pharmaceutical companies, and they are not eager to demonstrate that garlic is an effective and cheap alternative to their expensive antibiotics.

What is all but incredible about the germicidal powers of garlic is the fact of its uncanny selectivity: unlike ordinary antibiotics, which indiscriminately kill friend and foe alike -- I talked about that in connection with yogurt -- garlic destroys only the hostile germs but leaves the friendly ones alone. No need for supplementary yogurt if you attack an intestinal infection with garlic.

What to drink

Having been told in broad terms what to eat,

you may want to know what you can drink that is safe from the point of view of good health. After all, a ban has been pronounced on liquor, coffee, and soft drinks. What is there left to drink?

There are lots of things to choose from. However, before I give you the list of legitimate drinks, let me dispel a very common misconception -- that wanting a soft drink or a beer means being thirsty. If, offering a glass of water to a guest who has asked for a soft drink or a beer, you get a "No, thank you," it is pretty safe to assume that he is not thirsty in a physiological sense. If he were, he would readily settle for water. Water -- even warm water -- tastes good if one is really thirsty. What your guest experiences is a craving for a substance other than water -- caffeine and/or sugar in the soft drink, alcohol in the beer -- and he mistakes the craving for thirst.

Genuine thirst is the body's signal that it needs water -- water, not caffeine, sugar or alcohol. Water is needed for most of the thousands of biochemical processes that take place in the body at all times. Water serves moreover as the vehicle of transport for the movement of nutrients to, and of waste products from, the cells. Without water, life as we know it would not be possible.

The body constantly loses water -- through the kidneys (urine), the skin (sweat), the lungs (moisture in breath) and the feces. Water thus lost has to be replaced. In part it is replaced by food, especially fruit and vegetables, which consist largely of water. When food does not supply enough water to make up for lost fluid, your body lets you know that it needs more by making you feel thirsty. But, no matter what you drink, it is the water content of a beverage that matters.

In some of the things you drink -- green tea, certain herbal teas, vegetable and fruit juices -- the water comes enriched with extra nutrients (vitamins, mineral and, at least in fruit juices, enzymes); in others -- soft drinks, coffee, beer, etc. -- the water has been polluted by substances that are incompatible with wholesome living.

Don't, by the way, confuse so-called fruit drinks with genuine fruit juices. They come in cans, in cartons or in bottles. They come ready to drink, they come as syrups to be diluted, they come as crystals to be dissolved in water. Usually their names contain either the term "fruit" or the name of a particular fruit as in "orange drink" or "pineapple drink." But that's all many of them have in common with real fruit -- the name. The best of them consist of diluted fruit concentrate admixed with such additives as artificial coloring, artificial flavoring agents, chemicals to keep the preparations from fermenting and lots of sugar. The worst of them are mere synthetic imitations of the real thing. Hands off them even if the label says "Vitamin this or that added." If vitamins are indeed added, they are added in such minute quantities that one would have to drink gallons of the stuff to make a difference. But then the harm done by the undesirable additives would far outweigh the benefits of the desirable ones.

So, put <u>water</u> at the top of your list of desirable drinks. Apart from water, add those drinks to your list in which water comes enriched with extra nutrients or has at least not been polluted with undesirable ingredients.

Genuine fruit juices should be regarded as food rather than drink and handled accordingly. If someone living in Northern Nigeria tried to quench his thirst with nothing but fruit juice during the hot season, he would take in so many calories there would be little room for any other food. Think of fruit juices as a treat to reward yourself with rather than as drink.

Remember too that you are nutritionally better off eating the whole fruit than drinking only the juice. Moreover, if you eat the whole fruit you are much less likely to "overdose" than when you drink the juice.

Another legitimate drink is <u>surrogate coffee</u>. In Europe and in North America, natural food outlets sell various brands and blends of herbal coffee. The main ingredients are toasted grain and chicory, substances which deserve to be put on the positive side of the nutritional scale. But you can easily make your own surrogate coffee. Here is how:

Roast a little wheat or sorghum till it is dark brown. Just how dark is a matter of taste. Grind or pound it. Put some of the ground/pounded "coffee" into lightly boiling water -- try two tablespoons for half a liter of water -- and let it simmer for a few minutes. Remove it from the source of heat and let it steep for a few more minutes. Then strain and drink it, with or without milk. You will be surprised how much like real coffee it tastes. And it is nutritionally safe.

In Europe and in North America, herbal teas, another kind of legitimate drink, are sold at natural food outlets, at herbalists' and at delicatessens. Here are some of my own favorites: mint, chamomile, elderflower, lemon grass and sorrel (mauve). In Africa I always had a patch of mint in my garden. In Jeddah, where I had neither garden nor mint patch, I found fresh mint in the majority of supermarkets. Many spice stores carried dried sorrel. For all I know, there may be local varieties of herbal teas that I never even heard of.

Herbal teas are deliciously flavored, wholesome water. Some of them supply traces of minerals and/or vitamins. They can be taken hot or cold -- hot for breakfast, cold at any time a cold drink is desired. During the hot season, there should always be a pitcher of herbal tea in the fridge. Iced mint tea with a few drops of lime juice is a delicious drink for a hot day. So is a thin infusion of sorrel blossoms with a sprinkle of lemon juice. No need for sugar. Take my word for it: you quickly get used to drinking your herbal teas unsweetened. Green tea comes with an anti-oxidant complement, which many researchers believe protects against cancer.

Supplements

If circumstances were ideal -- if we had access to clean, mineral-rich water all the time; if our food were grown organically on soils rich in minerals; if our diets were truly balanced; if we, and our mothers and fathers, had always abstained from such substances as coffee, soft drinks, nicotine and alcohol; if we always had enough exercise -- there would probably be no need for supplements. However, circumstances being less than ideal for most people the world over, most of them would benefit from some supplementation. Since individual needs vary greatly, it is not possible to make universally valid recommendations. Nevertheless I can offer a basic list of those supplements which most people could be expected to benefit from.

<u>Vitamins A and D</u>: They usually come together in capsules of 5,000 IU of A and 400 IU of D. However 400 IU of D is little better than nothing. The human body produces its own Vitamin D if it gets sufficient exposure to sunlight. So during the summer months we may get enough Vitamin D from the sun. We certainly don't from October to April in our mid-latitude setting. That's why the majority of midlatituders are D deficient in winter with often disastrous consequences. Vitamin D is our best protection against infections of any kind, the flu included. Why do we get flu epidemics in winter but not in summer? Take 5000 IU during the winter months and forget about the flu and the flu shot. I have never had a flu shot. They'd have to tie me down to get one into me. Yet I don't remember ever having had the flu.

As for Vitamin A, 5000 to 10000 IU is a reasonable daily dosis. Liver, apricots, red peppers, carrots, spinach, mangoes and papaya are good food sources of Vitamin A. No need for supplementation if you consume these foods regularly.

<u>The B-vitamins</u>: He who regularly eats the B-rich foods -- brewer's yeast, wheat germ, liver, whole-wheat bread -- need not worry about his intake of the B's. Otherwise a good B-complex supplement would

be advisable, one that contains all the B's, not just a few of the cheaper ones. Here is the complete list of the known B's: B1, B2, B3, B6, B12, Pantothenic Acid, Folic Acid, Biotin, Choline, Inositol and Para-aminobenzoic Acid.

Vitamin C: I recommend at least 1000 mg a day, divided into three or four doses spread through the day. At times of great stress, requirements for Vitamin C go up. Keep in mind that excess of joy is as much a stress as is excess of sorrow. I take +/- 5,000 mg of C a day regularly. When I feel under great stress, I may take 10,000 mg or more in the course of a day. Good food sources of Vitamin C are oranges, limes, guavas, red peppers, papaya and potatoes.

Vitamin E: 200 to 400 IU is a reasonable daily dosis. If your blood pressure is high, you should consult a physician who is knowledgeable about Vitamin E. If that is not possible, start with very small doses of the vitamin, perhaps 30 IU a day. After a few weeks you can gradually increase the dosis by 20 or 30 IU a day till you have reached the desired dosis. Good food sources of Vitamin E are wheat germ, whole wheat, lettuce, peanuts and most unrefined vegetable oils.

Calcium: Here are some good food sources of calcium -- cheese, yogurt, milk, sesame seeds, spinach, blackstrap molasses and sardines.

Magnesium: It is important to note that calcium and magnesium are a team. The more you get of one, the more you need of the other. Since there are few common food sources of magnesium, people generally are more likely to be deficient in magnesium than in calcium. I reach for a magnesium supplement before reaching for a calcium supplement.

Zinc: I recommend 20 to 50 mg a day. Men approaching middle age should be particularly concerned about their zinc intake, for zinc is of vital importance for a healthy prostate. Zinc moreover forms part of many enzyme systems. It is essential for healthy skin and hair. Good food sources of the mineral are sardines, liver, egg yolk, whole wheat and ginger root.

These are the supplements I would not want to live without. If someone asked me to compile a list of supplements which might be counted on to slow aging and to help prevent the ills commonly associated with old age, that list would be much like my list of basic supplements.

Strategy 2: exercise A minimum of physical exercise is essential for good health. In the past, most people had more than enough physical exercise built into their daily routine: they walked long distances, they worked in the fields, they did by hand many of the things that are now done by machines. No need for them to introduce exercise artificially into their lives.

Times have altered. More and more people get less and less exercise. Things are worst in developed countries. There very few people get any exercise from their work any more. Just look at farming, which used to be one of the most labor-intensive occupations. From the preparation of the soil for planting right through to harvesting, everything is done by machines. Walking? People in developed countries don't walk any more. They walk from their homes to their cars, from their cars to their offices and back again. And they show it too: lots of them are fat and conspicuously out of shape.

Throughout North America the most popular sport is armchair athletics -- millions of non-athletes watching a few real athletes -- highly paid professionals most of them -- on TV. In much of the developed world physical effort is avoided like the plague. Once, while talking to a group of North Americans about the necessity of exercise, I pointed out the benefits of jogging. Quipped a typical representative of North American manhood: "I don't believe in that sort of self-inflicted torture."

Developing countries are catching up fast. There too more and more people are getting less and less exercise, even in the poorest of African countries. In the big urban centers, many people have their own cars, and most of the car owners go everywhere by car. Those who don't have cars go by taxi or by mini-bus. Only the poorest of the poor walk. And they dream of the day when they too will be able to afford mechanized transportation. Many people moreover spend much of their working time sitting in offices and much of their leisure time sitting in front of television sets. The human body is not meant for such a life of inactivity.

    Most of the students I taught in Saudi Arabia seemed to feel about walking up a few flights of stairs much as the American felt about jogging. My office was on the fourth floor of a five-story building. I, an old man of sixty-five then, always took the stairs going to my office, sometimes three and four times a day. Of the hundreds of students that frequented the building, all but a handful took the elevator. They took the elevator even if they wanted to go up only one floor. They thought me old-fashioned, if not simple-minded, for not wanting to ride in the elevator.

    Much educating needs to be done. People must be made to understand that a certain minimum of physical exercise is essential for building and maintaining good health. They must be made to understand that, if they do not get that minimum of physical exercise from their work, they have to introduce exercise artificially into their lives. Attitudes have to be reshaped. Many of my African acquaintances considered a life without physical effort the fulfillment of their dreams -- a car of their own so that they wouldn't have to walk, servants to do the physical work for them. The irony of it is that in this sort of setting the servants would be fit and healthy while the masters would end up out of shape and prone to illness.

    My African neighbors thought me a fool for doing what in their opinion was work for servants or for *junior* relatives -- carrying the groceries from the car to the house, carrying a bucket of water from the well to the house when the public water system failed to deliver, hoeing and weeding the garden, etc. They all subscribed to the viewpoint common among well-to-do Africans and typified by the man who told me, "What's the point of getting to a position where you can get others to do the physical work for you if you still do it yourself?" True, I would not want to be carrying water all day long. I have more productive activities to fill my time with. But carrying a bucket of water now and then means giving some of the many neglected muscles in my body a little exercise. It's all in the way you look at things. If you think carrying a bucket of water is an unpleasant chore, carrying a bucket of water will be an unpleasant chore. If you look at it my way, carrying a bucket of water -- or walking a few flights of stairs, for that matter -- can be fun even while it gives you a little much-needed exercise.

Exercise is for everybody. It is not just for the track star, for the soccer player, for the ballet dancer. It is not just for boys and men either. It is for women as well as for men; it is for the young, for people in their prime and for those who are past their prime. I know people who, though they are in their 80s, still take part in public fun runs.

If anything, older people need exercise *more* than young people, not less. Unfortunately most people become physically less active as they grow older. So their muscles lose their tone and their vigor, their digestive system becomes sluggish, their cardiovascular system deteriorates. At first they feel vaguely out of sorts: they do not sleep well, but when they are up and about, they tire easily; and they tend to put on weight. So they become physically even less active and in consequence tire even faster. A vicious cycle is complete.

Many old people become prey to degenerative diseases that affect the digestive tract (ulcers, diverticulitis, constipation), the cardiovascular system (atherosclerosis with attendant poor circulation and high blood pressure), the organs of elimination (kidneys, liver, lungs), etc. And everywhere both laymen and medical experts alike accept these infirmities as the inevitable accompaniment of growing old though lots of healthy old people the world over give them the lie, people who remain physically and mentally fit far into old age. The truth of it is that the infirmities commonly attributed to old age are really the cumulative wages of faulty living, above all lack of exercise. If they are more common in old age, it is precisely because they have had more time to develop. Every individual has it in his power to delay the onset of these infirmities through a wholesome lifestyle, a big part of which is regular exercise.

If the elderly cannot claim exemption from exercise, neither can women. In the West, many women don't exercise for fear that exercise will put bulky muscles on them and make them look like men. Their fears are altogether groundless. There is something in the hormonal make-up of women that keeps them from becoming muscular even if they exercise heavily. Just look at the millions of African women who pound grain all their lives. Their arms, strong though they are, retain their feminine contours.

So, ladies, the argument that exercise robs you of your feminine looks does not wash. At the same time, exercise has lots of positive effects that should be of interest to you. It firms sagging muscles; it makes loose flab disappear from the underpart of the upper arm; it trims the abdomen and it takes cellulite off the hips and the buttocks; it generally redistributes weight, taking it off where it should come off (the waist or the thighs) and putting it on where more weight is desirable (spindly legs). Women need not suspend exercise even during pregnancy. On the contrary, women who keep their bodies in good shape through regular exercise give birth more easily than women who are in bad physical shape. And chances are that they bear healthier babies.

From the point of view of good health, the most important single purpose of exercise is to (re)condition the cardiovascular system, i.e. the heart and the blood vessels. An efficient cardiovascular system performs well its two main functions -- that of supplying all parts of the body with nutrients and that of removing waste products from them. No matter how good your nutrition, you cannot hope to get the full benefit of it if your cardiovascular system is in bad shape; and if waste products are not removed efficiently from the countless cells of the body, the stage is set for disease.

Now, the term "exercise" covers a lot of ground. It includes weight-lifting and yoga, calisthenics and running, walking and swimming, and many other activities. While every form of exercise has something to recommend it to somebody, not every form of exercise can be relied on to keep one's cardiovascular system in good shape. Only one form of exercise does that -- aerobic exercise.

If exercise is to rate as aerobic, it must involve the whole body, or large parts of it, in vigorous movement. The cumulative effect of it must be to increase the work load of the heart so that its beat goes up by about 70%; that is to say, if your resting heart rate is 70 beats per minute, during aerobic exercise it should increase to about 120. And it should stay there for a very minimum of 15 to 20 minutes. Such forms of exercise as weight-lifting, calisthenics, stretching routines and the whole range of yoga movements and postures, excellent as they may be in their own right, do not qualify as aerobic because they do not represent a sustained and continuous effort. Here are some forms of exercise that do: walking, running, stationary running, bicycling, swimming, skiing, cross-country skiing, rowing, mountain climbing, rope skipping, and a good many games such as soccer (for all but the goalie), basketball, hockey and tennis.

The heart is a muscle. Like every muscle, it benefits from exercise. Like every muscle it needs exercise to become and to remain fit. Different muscles need different kinds of exercise. The exercise that is best for the heart is aerobic exercise.

Most people who get started on a program of aerobic exercise soon notice that their heart rate goes down. A slowing of about ten beats in the course of a few months is not uncommon. It is a good sign. It is an external manifestation of the heart's improving efficiency, a sign that it can now accomplish with fewer beats the task of sending the blood to the most distant parts of the body. That means less wear and tear for the heart and probably greater life expectancy for its owner.

Let me put this to you in mathematical terms. A heart rate of 50 beats per minute is nothing unusual for an aerobically fit adult. An aerobically unfit adult might have a heart beat of 75 beats per minute, fully 1/3 more. In the course of a year, this would work out to approximately 120 days less work for the fit heart. Imagine -- four months' holidays a year for the fit heart, while the unfit heart would have to slug it out all the way.

An American heart specialist maintains that he has never known of anyone capable of doing a marathon to die of heart problems. He believes that one's life expectancy is proportionate to the distance one is capable of running.

Apart from the over-all benefit of aerobic exercise -- that of (re)conditioning the cardiovascular system -- aerobic exercise recommends itself through a host of other benefits. One of them is that it makes you sweat, and sweating assists your body in ridding itself of metabolic waste.

Aerobic exercise is, moreover, good for the lungs. Most sedentary people are shallow breathers. They tend to take small breaths, which fill only a small part of their lungs. The rest of their lungs contains stale air, which gets exchanged only very slowly and incompletely. If you are a sedentary, non-exercise person, try taking a deep breath now -- as deep a breath as you can without actually straining. At the end of it you probably feel something akin to pain. Your lungs are not used to expanding and filling all the way. They are quite likely to have shrunk in actual size too owing to lack of exercise.

Aerobic exercise changes all that. It gets your lungs working all the way. It turns you into a deep breather, who fills his lung with air all the way and who exhales all the way. No more trapping of stale air in unused corners of your lungs. Eventually your lungs will regain their full efficiency in the exchange of gases. They will regain their optimal size.

These benefits -- improved cardiovascular fitness, the cleansing effect of sweating, better lungs and better breathing -- are the more immediately obvious benefits of aerobic exercise. There are many more, some of them not so readily obvious. In fact, after one has been on a regular aerobic exercise program for a while, all systems tend to work better. Every cell of the body benefits from improved cardiovascular fitness, which means better blood circulation and better oxygenation, and every muscle benefits from the massage effect of aerobic exercise. From head to toe, everything works better.

The brain works better. Brain cells respond more quickly to changes in oxygenation than most other cells. If they are starved of oxygen, they get sluggish, as they do in crowded rooms, where ventilation is inadequate. There, the combined breathing of too many people uses up more oxygen than is replaced. The oxygen content of the air goes down. Though people continue to breathe apparently normally, less oxygen enters their lungs with each breath. And the brain cells are among the first to be affected. Their owners feel drowsy. Some may pass out. Conversely, if brain cells are richly supplied with oxygen, they perform well. A cardiovascular system that is super-fit thanks to regular aerobic exercise gets lots of oxygen to the brain.

If the brain functions more efficiently with aerobic exercise, so do the senses. Sight, hearing, smell, taste and touch -- they all tend to become more acute with aerobic exercise.

Aerobic exercise puts new life into the internal organs. The digestive tract, for instance, responds with new vigor. People who have had a long history of constipation, suddenly find that they can do without laxatives. Even sex works better.

Aerobic exercise is good for the legs. Many sedentary people, who do not exercise regularly, develop leg problems -- leg cramps, which plague them especially at night in bed; diffuse pains in the legs, which radiate from the deep veins; and, the most serious of them all, thrombophlebitis (blood clots blocking the heartward flow of the blood and resulting in painful inflammation of the affected vein). People who perform aerobic exercise regularly are not likely to develop any of these problems; those who already have them can hope to rehabilitate their legs through gently graduated aerobic exercise.

Most leg problems have to do with the fact that venous blood does not easily return to the heart, especially from the lower limbs. In the upper parts of the body, the heartward flow of the venous blood is assisted by the pull of gravity. In the lower parts of the body, gravity impedes the return of the venous blood to the heart. In the lower extremities, it is largely the movement of contiguous muscles that "pumps" venous blood back to the heart. As muscles alternately contract and expand, they squeeze the veins embedded in them, and the blood contained in these veins is pushed heartward, as it were, since a system of successive one-way valves prevents it from escaping in the opposite direction. This pumping effect of the muscles is most pronounced during vigorous exercise.

Aerobic exercise is the ideal strategy of weight control. Crash diets do not work. Most of them are expensive, nutritionally disastrous and boring. For all these reasons and more, dieters cannot stay on them indefinitely. But if they stop, nine times out of ten they put the weight back on faster than they lost it.

The only sensible and lasting solution to the problem of weight control is aerobic exercise -- aerobic exercise combined with a truly wholesome diet.

In developing countries many people still believe that being fat is a sign of good health. I want to tell them emphatically that that's wrong. Being fat is not compatible with good health. A truly healthy person is never fat. In fact, being overweight is itself a sign that health is beginning to break down. So, if you are overweight, do something about it before the damage becomes irreparable.

There is another benefit of aerobic exercise, one that is of particular interest for people whose nerves are bad, people who feel tense and irritable, people who are prone to depression. The benefit I have in mind is the tranquilizing effect which aerobic exercise produces. When I get to feel tense or anxious or depressed -- it seems these things happen to the best of us -- I put on my running shoes and gently jog a few miles. It never fails: I return to my point of departure a different man. I feel relaxed, I feel cheerful and optimistic again. Probably a spin-off of this tranquilizing effect -- aerobic exercise can be relied on to relieve tension headaches.

I know of a psychiatrist in Canada who jogs with his patients. He maintains that many of them find jogging a wonderful antidote to anxiety and depression. A study carried out at the Biodynamics Laboratory of the University of Wisconsin showed that for some people aerobic walking is effective therapy even for migraine headaches, that most intractable of all headaches.

The mechanism of this tranquilizing effect is not understood very well. It probably has to do with the fact that aerobic exercise relaxes most of the body's muscles. Relax the muscles, relax the mind; relax the mind, relax the muscles. It may also have to do with certain chemical substances released into the blood during aerobic exercise. These substances, called endorphins, are similar to morphine and they act like small doses of morphine -- they deaden sensations of pain and they relax.

Whatever the cause of the relaxation effect of aerobic exercise, there is no doubting the effect itself. And the marvelous thing about it is that there are no undesirable side effects. What more can one ask for -- a very effective tranquilizer without nasty side effects. With the chemical tranquilizers used in Western Medicine the big problem is side effects. The side effects of some of them are worse that the ills they are supposed to cure. One of the worst side effects is that they are addictive.

One last benefit of aerobic exercise -- the cumulative effect of all the benefits listed and discussed -- it contributes to an over-all sense of well-being. Practice aerobic exercise for a few months and you will find that you feel better, more alive than you did before, that you feel more energetic, more vigorous. Friends will tell you that you look younger and better. And chances are that aerobic exercise will help you stay young longer.

I Have lately been performing a special variation of jogging – ***interval training***. It is something that can be adapted to any kind of aerobic exercise. Essentially it means alternating between high-intensity short bursts and longer periods of going at it easy. More specifically, having warmed up first with about five minutes of easy jogging, I do an all-out sprint of about 100 yards, slow down to easy jogging for two hundred yards, another burst of an all-out 100-yards sprint, etc. I do eight complete cycles of it and conclude with three to five minutes of a brisk walk to warm down. This I do every third day. During the intervening two days, I do 5 km of gentle jogging.

The most interesting benefit of interval training is the fact that it stimulates the body to produce human growth hormone again, one of the secrets of good health and long life. Go do a web search for "The benefits of interval training" to find out more.

A lifestyle that keeps you healthy is bound to keep you young. If you live so that you get ill, you obviously short-change your body in some way or other -- through nutritional sins, through lack of exercise, through lack of rest, etc. Parts wear out prematurely. Illness itself becomes a stress that consumes vital energy and contributes to aging.

Getting started. I hope I have convinced you that aerobic exercise is for you too, that in fact you cannot afford not to get started on aerobic exercise yourself. The next thing to do is show you how to get started and help you choose a form of aerobic exercise you can live with.

The most important piece of advice for the beginner is to get started slowly. Most people make the mistake of trying for too much too fast. When you are ready to get yourself started on a program of aerobic exercise, keep this in mind: no matter how little you do at first, it is a lot more than you have been doing. When I started jogging some forty years ago, I was desperately out of shape and about 40 pounds too heavy. The first few weeks were sheer hell, and it took all I had of angry determination to keep going. I made matters worse by doing what most beginners do -- I tried to get there too fast. For some time my feet were so sore in the morning that I had to work them gingerly for several minutes before I could walk normally. My whole body was an assortment of aches and pains, the wages of my impatience. I could have done myself serious harm, but fortunately I came out of the ordeal intact. If I had to do it again, I'd be much easier on myself and would probably get there faster.

With each variety of aerobic exercise discussed below, I give you an idea how much time you should spend to obtain the minimum of exercise value needed to get and/or keep your cardiovascular system in good working order. But don't take those figures as challenges to be met all at once. Think of them as something to work up to. At the beginning, rather than think that you should do so much in a given span of time, let your heart tell you how much or how little you should be doing. When you exercise, your heartbeat accelerates. That's normal. Once you are truly fit, it is virtually impossible to over-rev your heart. But, until you are truly fit, you should not push your heart past certain safe limits.

Here is a simple formula, age-adjusted, with which you can determine an exercise heart rate that is safe for you. Take 220 as a starting figure. Subtract your age from that. What's left represents your absolute maximum heart rate, something you should probably never try to reach, certainly not until you are superbly fit. Seventy percent of this never-to-be-reached maximum is your exercise rate.

Let's apply the formula to a real case -- my own. I am almost 80 years old. Therefore

220 - 80 = 140 bpm (absolute maximum)
70% of 140 bpm would be 98 bpm.

This 98 bpm is my target rate for regular exercise. Every now and then -- half a dozen times a month -- I put in a hard day. For the hard days I have a different target bpm -- 80 % of maximum, or +/- 112 bpm. To reach the hard-day target of about 115 bpm, I have to run faster and longer than for the regular 98 bpm. For you, the hard-day bpm, whatever it may be in your case, is prohibited until you are sure that you are reasonably fit. Till you are, stick to the 70% of maximum. It represents enough of a workload for your heart to get in shape; at the same time it is safe. At the end of my interval training, my heart rate approaches 140 bpm. But that's no cause for alarm. After some forty years of jogging and an otherwise healthy lifestyle, my heart can take it. I can confidently say, "If my legs can take it, my heart can."

If you are 40 and haven't exercised for some time, especially if you are a little overweight, you may be well advised to limit yourself to only 60% of maximum for perhaps a month. That would be 96 bpm.

One more safety regulation for the beginning aerobic exercise convert. Let him check the recovery rate of his heart. Five minutes after exercise, his bpm should be 20 to 25 beats lower than his target rate. Ten minutes after exercise, it should not be more than 90 bpm. If he finds his bpm higher at either point, he's asking too much of his heart. He'd better slow down.

Here is an easy way to check your bpm. Place index finger and thumb of your right hand against your wind pipe so that they come to rest one to the left and the other to the right of, and just behind, the Adam's apple. You will feel a strong pulse there. Look at a watch with a second hand or with a running counter of seconds and count the number of pulse beats for ten seconds. Multiply the figure thus obtained by six and you have your pulse bpm for that particular moment. Instead of the ten-seconds count, I prefer to count my pulse for 30 seconds and multiply the result by too. It is more accurate.

At first let yourself be guided by your heartrate rather than try to perform the minimum-exercise routines you'll find in Dr. Cooper's *Aerobics*. Borrow a copy from a library or buy one used for a buck or two from Amazon. In that book you will find schedules for any aerobic exercise readily available. For, if your heart is not in good shape, even Dr. Cooper's minimum exercise routines may push your bpm past the safe limit. Later, when you have rehabilitated your heart, those same routines -- far from overloading your heart -- may not be enough to raise your bpm to the target rate.

Keep this in mind too -- if you hope to rehabilitate your heart, you must exercise *regularly*. He who exercises only sporadically -- once this week, twice next week, not at all the week after -- may do himself more harm than good. He subjects his heart to the effort of exercise without ever giving it a chance to get into good shape.

Intervals between exercise sessions should not be longer than two days. Frequent exercise sessions of short duration are better than infrequent ones of long duration. If you are prepared to invest 105 minutes a week in jogging, you have the following options of scheduling those 105 minutes:

7 x 15.0 minutes	acceptable
6 x 17.5 minutes	better... you should have at least one day of rest
5 x 21.0 minutes	probably ideal
4 x 26.0 minutes	acceptable
3 x 35.0 minutes	would still do
2 x 53.0 minutes	not advisable
1 x 105.0 minutes	DON'T! Probably do more harm than good.

There remains the question of a medical check-up. If you have a history of cardiovascular problems -- high blood pressure, varicose veins, heart trouble, etc. -- a medical examination is a must before you get started on an aerobic exercise program; and, if at all possible, it should be done by a specialist. Even without a history of cardiovascular problems, a medical check-up is advisable if you are over 40, if you have not been active for more than half a year, especially if you are overweight. Chances are that your doctor will give you the go-ahead for your exercise program. But, even if he does, you should not let that lull you into a false sense of security. Unless your doctor practices aerobic exercise himself and is knowledgeable about the demands aerobic exercise makes on the heart, he may pronounce you fit when you aren't. Examining a heart at rest with a stethoscope, as most general practitioners do, says little about how that heart will respond under the stress of exercise. Better play it safe, medical or no medical: give your heart a chance to become fit before you challenge it with high-intensity performance.

Here is a list of activities that deserve to be called aerobic:

Stationary running	Rowing
Rope skipping	Swimming
Dancing	Skiing

Stair-climbing   Water skiing
Exercise machine Mountain climbing
Walking
Jogging

Walking and jogging, by the way, are merely different intensities of the same activity. The only significant difference is that you have to invest a little more time in walking to get the same exercise value as in jogging.

In addition, there are certain games which qualify as aerobic, provided they are played fairly vigorously and continuously, among them soccer, basket ball, hockey, badminton, tennis and ping-pong. Golf and volleyball do not qualify as aerobic, the former not being strenuous enough, the latter not being sufficiently continuous.

The varieties of exercise listed in the right column are not readily practicable for ordinary people while the ones in the left column are for everyone who has no disqualifying physical handicap. Let's look at them more closely.

There are first the at-home varieties of aerobic exercise -- rope skipping, stationary running, dancing and stair climbing. They are for people who, for one reason or other, can't or don't want to exercise outdoors. They are also the alternative for bad-weather days. You may choose one of them to the exclusion of all the others, or you may do several of them on a rotating schedule like the following:

Monday   rope skipping
Tuesday   dancing
Wednesday   stationary running
Thursday   rest
Friday   stair climbing
Saturday   stationary running
Sunday   rest

You may even do several of them during the same exercise session -- rope skipping for a few minutes, dancing for a few minutes, etc.

Rope skipping. You don't even need a rope for this kind of exercise. If you have one, by all means use it; but, if you don't, skip as you would with a rope, arms going through the motion of swinging the rope while the legs do the skipping. Here is what a minimum exercise schedule according to Dr. Cooper would look like:

Skips per Minute	Time in minutes	Times per week	Total time
100 – 110	15	6	90
110 – 120	12	6	72
120 - 130	12	5	60

At first you will find it difficult, if not impossible, to skip for 12 minutes continuously. Take it easy. For the first month or so, do your 12 or 15 minutes by installments -- skip for 2 minutes (or until your calves tell you to stop), walk up and down for perhaps half a minute, skip for another two minutes, etc.

Stationary running. Some people refer to stationary running as "carpet jogging." It is running/jogging on the spot. To get the full training effect, your feet should come off the floor at least 8 inches with each running step. As with ordinary jogging, you can go faster or slower, earning accordingly more or fewer points in a given period of time.

Dancing. If dancing turns you on more than the other varieties of indoor exercise, dance your way to fitness. But you must move vigorously. A slow shuffle as in a tango or a slow waltz won't give you much of any training effect. Let your heart be your guide. If you keep your bpm at or near 60 % of maximum, you'll have to put in at least 20 minutes five times a week. At 70 % of maximum, do 20 minutes four times or 15 minutes five times a week. And keep in mind that I am talking only about the very minima of effort.

Stair climbing: If you have a flight of stairs in your house, walking/jogging up and down that flight of stairs is a good way to build and/or to maintain fitness. Of course climbing those stairs does you no good aerobically if you do it once up, once down at a time, as one does routinely in a house with stairs, though you should do so several times in the course of a day. To earn aerobic fitness points, you have to keep at it continuously for perhaps half an hour.

If there are no stairs to climb in your house, you can simulate stair climbing by stepping up and down a single step 7 to 8 inches high or a chair 15 to 18 inches high. You step up with one foot, then bring up the other foot; you step down with one foot (usually the one that stepped up first), then with the other, one at a time, no jumping. You'll find more precise information as to how much you should do to qualify for a minimum of fitness points in Dr. Kenneth Cooper's excellent book ***Aerobics.***

Exercise bike: If you can get your hands -- oops, should have said *feet*, not **hands** -- on an exercise bike, you can cycle your way to fitness without ever leaving your home. But I cannot give you a minimum schedule for the bike. One would have to make a different schedule for each one of the many makes of bike sold. At any rate, a set of instructions is usually supplied with a bike. That set of instructions should enable you to work out a minimum schedule of your own. Don't forget to watch your bpm when you work out your schedule.

So much for the at-home varieties of aerobic exercise. Let us now look at the three outdoor varieties which are readily practicable almost anywhere -- bicycling, walking, jogging.

The first two recommend themselves to many people by being "respectable." In my African setting, even the principal of the college where I taught could afford to appear in public on a bicycle and his Excellency the Bishop of Maiduguri could go for long walks. The two of them would not have wanted to be seen jogging in public. But these two types of exercise have the disadvantage that one must invest more time in them to get one's aerobic points.

Take the bicycle. Thanks to the operation of the wheel, it enables you to cheat gravity. On a bike you can move loads several times your own weight over considerable distances with relatively little effort. To do a mile on a bike requires much less effort than to walk a mile. True, going uphill on a bike may require more energy than walking uphill, but then going downhill requires no energy at all. And any bicycle route that has ups must have downs if the cyclist is to get back to his point of departure. From an aerobic point of view, on a route where short ups and downs alternate, the downhill parts so nearly cancel the uphill parts that very little, if any, training effect occurs. A training effect occurs only if the uphill parts are so long, or the cyclist peddles so hard, that his heart has no chance to return to normal during the descent. Ordinarily, therefore, one has to invest a fair bit of time in cycling in order to earn one's fitness points.

Much the same is true of walking. A leisurely stroll earns you no fitness points even if you are out for an hour. You have to walk briskly if you are to earn any aerobic fitness points at all. Even then you have to invest a lot of time. Let's assume you are prepared to walk three miles. If it takes you more than an hour to do the three miles, you earn few fitness points. If you do the three miles in 45 to 60 minutes, you have to put in at least six such three-mile walks a week to obtain the minimum exercise effect. Should you want to go out only five times a week, you would have to do the three miles in around 40 minutes. But that is faster than most people can walk. To obtain your basic exercise needs from walking, at a pace that can still be considered a walk, you'd have to do 4 miles in 60 to 80 minutes four times a week. But that adds up to a total of between 4 and 5 hours a week, more time than a good many people would be willing to invest in exercise.

Biking is not much better. To obtain the basic minimum of aerobic training, at a pace manageable for ordinary mortals, you'd have to do 8 miles in 35 to 45 minutes four times a week. That comes to a total of 2 1/2 to 3 hours.

However, if you chose jogging as your main exercise, 1 to 1 ½ hours spaced through the week would do it. Jogging, that is, you'd have to invest considerably less time than you would if you were to walk or to cycle to get your very minimum of fitness points. I would not want to settle for the minimum..

Surely you could spare that much time for exercise. If you think you can't, you may eventually have to spend much more time being sick

This is one of the reasons why I chose running as my form or exercise -- that it gives me more fitness points in less time than any other aerobic exercise readily available to me. I do other things occasionally: I go for long walks; I go swimming or cycling; I play a vigorous game of table tennis; on a bad-weather day, I may opt for one of the indoor varieties of exercise -- rope skipping, stationary running or stair climbing. But I do these things in addition to, not in place of jogging.

Now jogging may not appeal to you. You may consider jogging socially unacceptable. Lots of people in Canada, in Africa and in Saudi Arabia have told me that they could not face the ridicule their neighbors would heap on them if they started to run in public. I know what they mean. I have myself been laughed at many times, have been the butt of jokes on several continents. I remember a Spaniard at an outdoor cafe jeering, loud enough for all the guests assembled there to hear and to share the joke, "What are we going to do with it, catch it or shoot it?" He probably thought I would not understand. But, I have grown a thick skin. Let the fools laugh. I won't let their fatuous contempt keep me from doing what I consider one of the most important things in my life.

When I first started to jog in Africa in 1980, I was a sensation. People dropped whatever they were doing to gawk at the "bature" who had seemingly taken leave of his senses -- grown-up man with more than a little gray in his beard running for no apparent reason -- not running from danger, not running to catch something, just running. I found out later that my apparel -- a pair of shorts and a pair of running shoes -- was just more evidence to them that I was mad. In the villages near Maiduguri, which I explored jogging, my appearance caused pandemonium. Children screamed in fright and dashed for the safety of the nearest compound. Most women too, though they did not scream, took off as though they had seen a ghost.

Much has happened in Nigeria since. In 1985, the Federal Military Government of Nigeria urged all state governors to promote jogging in their jurisdictions. In Maiduguri, the capital of Borno State, Major General Waziri, then military governor of the state, launched a jogging club. Several thousand people watched him, accompanied by everyone of rank and name in the state, jog one lap around the track of the Police Grounds. Many more people watched the launching on television. And for many months after that, every Saturday morning, some of the most prominent citizens of Maiduguri could be seen jogging there. Now and then the governor himself turned up for a few laps. All that went a long way towards making jogging respectable in Nigeria, at least in the bigger cities.

Out in the country it was a different story. There jogging had not "arrived" by the time I left Nigeria, several years later. I remember jogging in a small village in Gongola State a few weeks before I left. A dignified-looking, old man stopped me with outstretched arms. "Tsoho," he asked me, "menene wannan gudu?" (Old man... what's the meaning of this running?) In my inadequate Hausa I tried to tell him

"Motsa jiki akwai amfani." (Exercise is good for you.) He was not impressed. In the tone of a teacher reprimanding a wayward student, he gave me to understand that it was not right for a "tsoho" like me to be running around like a little boy. Much to the amusement of the crowd that had gathered around us, he demonstrated to me how a "tsoho" should move about -- a stately walk, no faster than perhaps 2 km an hour, head held high, eyes looking straight ahead. I thanked him and resumed my jogging. When I looked back a few seconds later, I saw him shake his head in apparent displeasure. Now, if I were an inhabitant of that place, I don't know whether I would have the nerve to go jogging in the face of such massive disapproval. I would probably switch to a version of aerobic exercise that would be either less conspicuous or more acceptable.

I said above that I have chosen jogging as my form of aerobic exercise because it gives me more fitness points in a given span of time than any other form of exercise readily available to me. But that's only one of the reasons. Let me point out a few more. One of them is the fact that jogging, apart from what it does for my cardiovascular system, exercises most of the muscles of my body. As long as I jog, I don't really need any other kind of exercise. Feet, legs, behind, abdomen, chest, arms -- most of the muscles of all the major parts of my body get enough of a work-out through jogging to maintain good tone and general strength.

Something else that I like about jogging is that it is cheap and uncomplicated. No need to buy expensive equipment. A pair of running shoes and a pair of shorts is all you need. Flashy jogging suits are for the beginner or the Sunday jogger, who feels a need to call the world's attention to the fact that he is jogging. Veteran joggers are seldom seen in them. No admission fees for swimming pools or club membership fees. No expenses, no time wasted getting to and from your theater of action. Your theater of action is always where you are. You can step into it from your front door, and you can time your run so that the end of it gets you back to your point of departure. You can jog any time you feel like jogging, no need to synchronize your schedule with the opening times of a gymnasium or a swimming pool, no need to wait for partners or team mates....

Jogging moreover means constantly changing scenery, something you don't get when you exercise at home. I usually run early in the morning. I like to watch the world come alive. I run whichever way "the wind blows me," always curious what may meet my eyes around the next corner. I run in my own neighborhood and I run away from home. I have run in Mexico City, Vancouver and Montreal; in Madrid, London and Berlin; in Riyadh, Hong Kong and Manila; in Kano, Niamey and Timbuktu. Jogging is the ideal mode of locomotion for sight seeing: you cover a lot of ground, much more than you would walking, and you are very mobile, much more so than in a car -- you can go up one-way streets in the wrong direction, you can zoom along pedestrian or bicycle paths, you can cross parks and you can run in cemeteries. Any time you come to a spot that invites you to stay awhile, you can pull up without having to worry about where to park or what to do with your bicycle.

I like to run errands while I am out jogging. A message to be delivered, a letter to be mailed, a question to be asked -- things that would mean extra trips by car -- I do them while I am out jogging. I'd be out anyway, and since jogging is an anywhere exercise, I might as well run to the post office as anywhere else.

What I said earlier about the tranquilizing effect of aerobic exercise in general is true of jogging in particular. Talk to any veteran jogger who does more than the basic minimum of jogging about the "jogger's high" and he'll wax eloquent. He will tell you that now and then, when out on a longer run, he experiences something akin to euphoria, a sensation not unlike the pleasurable, heady feeling which sometimes follows the first few sips of a cup of tea when your stomach is empty and your reserves of energy are low. He will talk about altered states of consciousness, about communion with the deeper layers of self not accessible in the ordinary state of awareness, the layers where, among other things, creativity lodges. Would that words could substitute for experience! You, who have not experienced the jogger's high, find it difficult to attach meaning to his words. "Mind," you hear him say, "seems to slip out of focus so that lines of accustomed thought blur, vanish; new lines form to become either wholly new ideas or simply new ways of looking at old problems." He will tell you that he gets his best ideas during those moments of "high."

  I myself deliberately capitalize on those altered states of consciousness: I take "problems" with me when I go jogging. It may be a personal problem, which I have attacked in vain with the resources of the conscious mind; it may be a writing problem -- some recalcitrant passage which I have sweated over, biting my pen and going in circles; it may be a teaching problem -- how best to teach a certain item of English Grammar, etc. I take these problems with me hoping that the creative mood will descend on me during my run. And quite often they sort themselves out as if by magic.

  I don't experience the jogger's high unless I jog for 45 minutes or more. Even then it does not always happen. It cannot be predicted and it won't be bidden. But when it does come, it is a marvelous experience. And no price to pay in terms of a hang-over or other side effects.

  The irony of it is that this most pleasurable side effect of jogging is only for the initiated, those who are already sold on jogging and who can jog long enough to experience it. The uninitiated, those who need to be wooed for jogging to become fit, are barred from experiencing it precisely because they are not fit -- not fit enough to jog far enough to experience it.

I sometimes get to hear comments like "I wish I had your energy! If I did, I would be out there jogging too." People who think and say such things look at the situation through the wrong end of the telescope. I tell them that I do not run because I have energy; I have energy because I run.

Get this too: it is virtually never too late to get started. No matter how old you are, as long as there is enough life in you to get up from your chair and to walk to the end of the hall, you can be reclaimed. The old Latin saying "*Dum spiro, spero*," is literally true in this context: as long as you breathe, there is hope -- hope to be reclaimed.

The important thing is that you get off your behind and start walking, jogging, dancing or whatever it is you choose as your form of aerobic exercise. Don't rationalize. Don't say "I am in such bad shape that, if I should start to jog, I would collapse," and be content with being in bad shape. For, if you don't exercise, your bad shape will worsen, no doubt about it. Rather say "I *am* in bad shape. Time I did something about it." Only, don't forget to get started gently so as to give your out-of-shape heart a chance to revive. However, once your heart has been rehabilitated and is truly fit, it is virtually impossible to damage it by exercising too hard, provided the exercise is regular. Other parts of your body would pack it in long before your heart.

Strategy 3: adequate rest All of life's activities require energy. There are the obvious ones such as standing, walking, running; there such less obvious ones as the beating of the heart, the digestion of food, the removal of waste; there are such activities as thinking, emotional responding and dreaming; and there are activities which are quite beyond the limits of our conscious awareness, like the growing of new cells, the biochemical processes that occur in the liver, etc.; . To the man of medicine or the biologist, all these "activities" are stress, the term to be understood as meaning anything that makes demands on a person's reserves of energy. Some of the stresses go on even while we are asleep. As long as there is life, there is stress. Complete cessation of stress means death. The difference between the waking and the sleeping state is that in the former more energy is consumed than the body can generate while in the latter the body generates more energy than is consumed. Awake we get tired sooner or later; asleep we rest.

During periods of rest the body repairs the damage done by the stresses of living -- it eliminates toxic waste, it rebuilds damaged tissues and it generally replenishes the depleted reserves of energy. The more stress an individual is subject to, the more rest (s)he needs.

When we talk of stress in everyday life, we usually think of negative or unpleasant experiences such as too much pressure at work, worries, grief or fears. But pleasurable experiences are stress too. They too consume energy. Physical work is stress, but so is play. Intense concentration is stress whether it occurs during an examination or during a game of chess. Boredom is stress, but so is excitement. Grief is stress, but so is joy. People have died from an excess of grief, but they have also died from an excess of joy. The cumulative effect of stress is that we get tired.

In physiological terms, getting tired means several things. It means that the reserves of energy-producing carbohydrates are depleted. It means that waste accumulates in the cells. It means that cells and groups of cells get worn. To repair the damage -- replenish stores of energy, eliminate metabolic waste, repair worn tissues -- the body needs rest. If it does not get enough rest, it falls behind in its chores and eventually disease results.

Rest is, of course, a relative concept. The runner who is winded after a 6-minute mile recovers during a subsequent 9-minute mile. A tennis player rests when he sits down between games. The reader who, having read a suspenseful story, sits back closing his eyes, rests. However the only perfect form of rest is sleep.

Adequate rest is probably as important for good health in the long run as are the other strategies. Just what is adequate, the individual himself must determine, taking into account such things as the stresses he is subjected to, his personal health status, his individual needs of sleep, etc.

Strategy 4: relaxation Let there be a relaxed mind in a relaxed body. A relaxed body-mind ensemble is much less vulnerable to disease than one that is tense. There are certain activities which promote relaxation. Some of them will be examined in this section.

Most of the things modern man has come to regard as relaxation are really stresses in disguise -- smoking, a game of bridge or poker, television, the cinema, a party, etc. Genuine relaxation invigorates while the false varieties tire and enervate.

Genuinely relaxing activities are too quiet and uneventful to tempt modern man -- a leisurely stroll in the early morning air, playing a musical instrument, gardening, yoga, meditation -- he has no time for these, most of his time being taken up by the louder activities which high-powered advertising pushes on him.

Individual differences play a part. What is relaxation to one man may be a source of irritation to another -- listening to or playing a Mozart minuet, for example, or an hour of angling, or assembling a model airplane or knitting a sweater. But there are certain activities which work for everyone willing to perform them.

Exercise is one such activity, especially aerobic exercise. Many people think of exercise as something that tires. It can tire, no doubt, if one overdoes it. If, however, one stays well within one's limits, exercise invigorates and relaxes. Aerobic exercise, as I explained in the chapter on exercise, is a marvelous tranquilizer, one that has no undesirable side effects. If, when I begin to feel tense or when a touch of depression steals over me, I can find the time to don my running shoes to jog a few miles, I come back a different man -- relaxed, my optimism restored.

There are two special techniques of relaxation, which the great majority of people in the western world have only the vaguest notion of -- yoga and meditation. They deserve a closer look.

I used to think that to learn <u>yoga</u> I would have to enroll in a formal yoga course. That did not appeal to me and so for a long time I just thought about yoga now and then but did not get down to doing it. Gradually, however, as I became better informed about health and healthful living, I picked up bits of information about yoga here and there, became more interested in it, and finally decided to find out what it was and what it could do for me. So I bought some books on yoga and worked my way through them. When I had finished, most of the fog had cleared. Here is a brief summary of what I learned:

1. No need for formal instruction. With a good book, you can teach yourself yoga in your own living room.
2. There is much more to yoga than standing on your head. Standing on your head is but one of many poses, which you may ignore if either you don't like or cannot do it.
3. You may ignore any pose that you do not like and select for your routine the ones you like. A little yoga is better than no yoga.
4. No need for the western obsession with perfection. As long as you do a yoga pose as well as you can, you will benefit from it.
5. Certain breathing exercises are part of yoga. They are beneficial for the body and for the mind.

With yoga, as with so many things, the proof of the pudding is in the eating. Give it a try for a few weeks and you may find yourself hooked on it. The benefits of yoga are numerous for him who practices it regularly. Among other things, yoga loosens stiff joints and relaxes tense muscles; it gently stimulates blood circulation, and an improved blood circulation, together with breathing exercises, results in better oxygenation of all the body's parts, particularly the brain; yoga relieves indigestion, constipation, insomnia, headaches and many other aches and pains; it gently massages vital organs and leaves them in better working order; a general improvement in body tone and in mental alertness gradually leads to a better self-image and to a more optimistic outlook on life.

    For the beginner, I recommend Kareen Zeebroff's *ABC of Yoga*. It contains 46 relatively easy yoga poses and four breathing exercises. It offers clear instructions, is easy to follow, and has photographs with each pose to illustrate the various stages of it. In time he can graduate to Kareen's second book, *Advancing with Yoga and Nutrition*.

    <u>Meditation</u> has, as it were, <u>come out</u>. One no longer has to hide it as though it were something unclean or politically suspect. And most people, though they may have had no personal experience of meditation, are at least familiar with the term "meditation." Nevertheless, a good many people still have curious ideas about it. For their sake, let me point out first what meditation is <u>not</u>, to clear the air the better to understand what it is.

    To begin with, meditation is not a religious rite or ritual. Though many people who are deeply religious practice meditation -- in the Christian tradition, the equivalent of meditation is contemplation -- one does not have to be religious, or for that matter believe in god or devil, to meditate. Further, meditation requires no special equipment: one does not need incense to meditate; one needs no crystal ball, no fetish, no holy water; one needs no drugs to get into the meditative state. On the contrary, meditation has itself freed many young people from drug addiction, and more and more of them discover that they can get "high" naturally on meditation itself.

Nor is meditation just silly kid or adolescent stuff. Very serious adults have practiced meditation in the past, and many cool-headed scientists or businessmen have adopted it in our era as a technique that enables them to cope better with the stresses of their respective situations.

When I mention meditation, people often ask me, "Well, when you meditate, just what do you meditate about?" This question, it seems, is prompted by the fact that the term "meditate" denotes both "to think intensely about something" and "to practice a technique of physical and mental relaxation." The questioner assumes that the two meanings are interchangeable. But they are not connected in any other way than that they happen to be lodged in the same word. In fact, *to **meditate*** in the sense under discussion means, as much as that is possible, not to think about anything at all.

Meditation, finally, is no more the monopoly of any one school of thought than salvation is the monopoly of any one religion. The partisans of TM (Transcendental Meditation) would have it that there is only one true school of meditation -- theirs. Nothing against TM -- the technique is good, and TM teachers usually teach it well; but one does not need to invest $ 300 in a TM course in order to learn how to meditate. Allan Watts's ***Meditation*** or LeShan's ***How to Meditate*** will do it. So will the following directions:

1. Pick a time and a place where you will not be disturbed for half an hour ... a reasonably quiet place, if possible.
2. Sit on a couch or in an easy-chair. Wriggle yourself into a comfortable position. Place your hands loosely beside your thighs or in your lap.
3. Once you feel physically comfortable, get yourself mentally comfortable. How? By being as passive as you can. Stop "trying." Just let things happen. You

do not even have to believe in meditation. As long as you don't sit there worrying whether it will work for you, it *will* work.

4. Step 4 differs from school to school. Several variations will be given below. The novice may try them all and eventually settle for the one that works best for him.

Variation 1: Close your eyes. Slowly take a deep breath and as slowly exhale. Now shift your attention from whatever is in your mind to your breathing. If your thoughts put up a fight, if they refuse to exit from the stage of your awareness, which has been undisputedly theirs all your life, simply ignore them and go on paying attention to your breathing. In no time at all there will be peace upstairs. After you have observed yourself breathe for the duration of a dozen breaths or more, you may attach a pair of syllables to each breath; e.g., the syllable <u>one</u> as you breathe in and the syllable <u>two</u> as you exhale. You may either think or softly mumble these syllables. The main purpose of this procedure is to help you break away from your normal pattern of thought.

  Basically one of two things may happen -- the meditator either loses himself completely in a state of mind that is not conscious of itself or of anything else, or he becomes conscious of certain thoughts -- the fact, for instance, that he is punctuating each breath with the syllables <u>one</u> & <u>two</u>, the fact that he has stopped paying attention to his breathing, the fact that he is trying to meditate, etc. The state of mind which is not aware of itself or of anything else is the state he wants to be in. Paradoxically, the moment he knows that he is in it, he is not longer in it; for then he has become conscious again. However, when he does become conscious, all he needs to do is return to his point of departure; that is, think or mumble <u>one-two</u> again, as he feels his breath enter and leave his lungs. In no time at all he will lose himself again. A third thing may happen -- he may drift off to sleep. No cause for concern, unless he oversleeps his lunch hour and does not get back to work on time. Until he is fairly certain that he will not fall asleep and miss his next appointment, it may be a good idea for him to set a timer. Otherwise, all he needs to do when he becomes aware that he must have fallen asleep is calmly to take note of it and to return to his point of departure. He may meditate for about twenty minutes. Then he should slowly move his arms and his legs and stretch his whole body. After opening his eyes, he should sit for a few more seconds and then get up slowly, ready to step back into the routine of his day. He will feel wonderfully refreshed.

Variation 2: Instead of focusing on his breathing, the meditator may focus his attention on a pleasant sense object -- a flower, a lit candle, the picture of a person dear to him, etc. He should not think <u>about</u> the object. He should simply let his eyes come to rest on it, to the exclusion of other things, and confidently allow matters to develop. He should breathe normally through his nose. If conscious or semi-conscious thoughts clamor for his attention, he should simply refuse to entertain them. If, as he continues to look at his object, his eyes should feel the least bit of fatigue, he should gently permit them to close. That's all. If he becomes conscious, he should return to his point of departure. After about twenty minutes, he may come out of meditation as in Variation 1 above.

Variation 3: This time the aid for breaking away from conscious thought is a sound -- a mantra. Devotees of TM will warn you that no mantra will work except one assigned to you in a personal interview by a trained teacher of TM. A mantra so assigned will of course work, but so will any sound the meditator finds pleasant and soothing. It may be a single syllable, a word, a phrase or a whole sentence. It may be a sound with meaning or a sound without meaning. I for one like the sound Allan Watts uses -- ahm ... ahmmmm ...

ahmmmmmmmm .... The meditator may chant it softly at various pitches till he hits the pitch that "turns him on." He may softly hum or intone the sound at that pitch for a minute or two and then let it fade, continuing however to hold an image of it in his mind as he did with the candle flame or the flower. If he becomes conscious of having lost the sound, he need only return to his point of departure.

Variation 4: This is the way of "getting there" that I use when I feel tense. It consists of two phases -- one that relaxes the body and one that relaxes the mind. For the body part, the meditator lies on his back, legs slightly apart. To start with, he shakes his body loose and wriggles himself into a comfortable position. Then he thinks himself through a routine of relaxing his body part by part. He starts with his toes. To become fully aware of them, he gently tenses the muscles in them for a few seconds. Then he relaxes them and "forgets" about them as though they were no longer there. Next he "concentrates" on his feet. He gently turns them left and right, till he has the full feel of them. Then he lets go and forgets about them. Thus he slowly works his way up his whole body -- legs, thighs, behind, etc. By the time he gets to his scalp, his whole body is so completely relaxed that he is hardly aware it exists. To conclude this phase, he mentally sweeps over his body once more, this time without moving a muscle, without tensing a tendon. He starts with his toes, and in one continuous slow sweep he passes over his body thinking to himself: "Toes ... legs ... knees ... thighs ...so wonderfully relaxed I cannot feel they are there ... behind ... belly ... chest, shoulders ....

    To relax his mind, he first wipes away all conscious thought. If he misses a few scraps of thought with the first sweep of the mental eraser, he does not trouble to sweep again; they will soon disappear by themselves. Next he fetches from his memory files a place or a scene that is ringed with pleasant memories -- the hammock in his grandfather's back-yard, a friend of his and he in a boat at sunset, a hide-out among the rocks by the sea -- and he projects that place or scene on his inner screen. He savors the pleasant memories that surround it. Otherwise he treats it much like the candle flame or the flower after he has closed his eyes. It becomes a vehicle of departure. About twenty minutes later he returns to everyday reality as in Variation 1 above.

A few points to remember. These directions will get the novice there. If he wants more detailed instructions, he may read the chapter "The HOW of Meditation" in *How to Meditate*. The thing he must not do when he sets out to meditate is TRY to meditate. The only thing he may consciously do is direct his thoughts to his breathing, to the candle flame, the flower, or the mantra, and then "get out of the way." Whatever happens is good, as long as he does not try to make things happen. Whenever he becomes conscious of any mental activity – whether it is a thought his mind has been chasing or even the fact that he is meditating – he should detach himself and return to his point of departure. And – he should meditate regularly.

Meditation is credited with many positive effects on the meditator's physiology, his brain-wave activity, his ability to concentrate, etc. It relaxes body and mind. It is the most effortless of all the strategies. It is cheap. All it costs is a little of one's time. And it has no harmful side effects. So -- no risks, but much to gain.

Strategy 5: cleanliness Cleanliness is not merely a cosmetic matter. It is one of the strategies that are vital to good health. In our sense, cleanliness means keeping the body clean by means of clean water. It has nothing to do with the use of antiperspirants and other cosmetics, and very little if anything with the use of soap.

A great many North Americans have rather different views of cleanliness. They use soap much too liberally. They do so in the belief -- largely the result of soap advertising -- that one does not qualify as clean unless one also smells clean. That's what sells soap in North America -- its smell, not its cleansing properties. Virtually all toilet soaps sold in North America are highly scented. The better you smell after a shower, the cleaner you are.

Genuine cleanliness is characterized by the absence of smell, good or bad, not by the "Lux" or "Joy" smell. All a healthy body needs to achieve that state is clean water. Most soaps, moreover, are more likely to do harm than good. On one hand they tend to destroy the natural acid mantle of the skin, an important part of the skin's defense system against microbial invaders. On the other hand, especially when used in areas like the armpits or the groins, they weaken or destroy the native flora and thereby achieve the exact opposite of what's intended: an armpit that has had its ecology interfered with becomes prey to hostile microbes, which break down the inevitable sweat in ways that are accompanied by unpleasant odor. A vicious cycle is initiated. Because there is body odor -- euphemistically referred to as BO -- more soap is used; more soap sets the stage for more BO

Probably worse than the obsession with soap is the North American preoccupation with antiperspirants. Millions of North Americans have been conditioned to believe that, unless they treat their armpits with deodorant-antiperspirants, they are not "clean" enough to appear in human company.

One who takes cleanliness in the naturopathic sense seriously uses soap sparingly -- mainly to remove dirt that does not readily yield to water alone. For regular washing he uses nothing but water. As for antiperspirants, he would not so fly in the face of nature as to want to stop one of the principal functions of the skin -- sweating, not even in so small an area as the armpit. He would want to promote rather than to curb it.

Two aspects of cleanliness deserve notice. One of them is the washing of hands. Hands should be washed before handling food, whether it be the preparation or the eating of it, to avoid ingesting contaminants (organic or inorganic), which hands have plenty of opportunity to pick up in their routine of touching. Hands should be washed, food handling or not, after every visit to the toilet, particularly after a visit to a public toilet.

The rest of the body should be kept clean mainly to ensure that the skin can perform efficiently its two main functions -- the secretion of sweat and respiration. In the sweat, the body eliminates significant amounts of waste matter. Some of this waster matter stays behind when the fluid part of sweat evaporates. Unless it is washed off regularly, it clogs the pores of the skin and interferes with the free secretion of new sweat.

The skin's contribution to total respiration is considerable; it is, in fact, so great that the individual who should lose it would be doomed to die. Medical history records cases of child actors who died because, to represent angels on stage, they had their whole bodies painted with gold paint. The paint eliminated the skin's part of respiration and the victims died. Now, not washing waste residues off the skin does not cause immediate death, but it reduces the skin's respiratory capacity and thereby detracts from health.

Strategy 6: an occasional fast Fasting is at least as old as man's recorded history. For thousands of years it has played a part both in religious ritual and as a technique of healing. As a technique of healing it is still widely practiced in many parts of the world. It is only in North America, really, that the majority of medical men pooh-pooh it as dangerous faddism. But even in North America there are some doctors who endorse it. One of them is Doctor Allan Cott, a New

York psychiatrist of international renown. He recommends fasting unreservedly as the ultimate therapy for many of man's ills. His two books on fasting (see bibliography) are both informative and interesting.

There are various kinds of fasts. There is the absolute fast -- no food of any kind, no water. This is the fast practiced by Muslims the world over during the month of Ramadan. And there are modified fasts -- no food for a certain length of time but water, no food except fruit juices and water, no food except fresh, raw fruit and/or vegetables and water. Which type of fast you choose depends on what you want to accomplish. The kind of fast most commonly recommended for therapeutic purposes -- the kind Dr. Cott deals with in his two books -- means total abstention from food, solid or liquid, for a certain number of days, but liberal consumption of water; in fact, water should be drunk generously on this type of fast. "Days" here means periods of twenty-four hours, not just the hours of daylight. In this context, a one-week fast means no food at all for one week, neither during the hours of daylight nor at night.

The very idea of going without food for more than a few hours frightens many people in North America and Europe. All too many of them believe that, if they did not have their three square meals a day, they would feel weak and could not do their work efficiently, if at all. But from volumes and volumes of literature, old and new, that have been written about fasting, it is evident that fasting is perfectly safe for most people, and that all but a very few can fast safely for several weeks and come away from the fast healthier and more energetic than they were before it. However, no layman should undertake a "therapeutic" fast of more than two or three days' duration without the supervision of a doctor who is competent in monitoring a prolonged fast. And no one should undertake even a short "therapeutic" fast without informing himself first about fasting itself and about the right way to break a fast. Someone who has fasted for say seven days -- that is, has not eaten any food at all for seven days -- can do himself harm if he does not break his fast the right way.

Seven days without food is by no means the limit. I remember the story of a small plane carrying its pilot and a passenger that crash-landed somewhere in northern Canada a good many years ago. The two survived the crash-landing and until they were found, a month later, they lived on nothing but water -- water obtained from the snow they had landed in. The doctors who examined them were amazed at their good state of general health. Some Irish hunger strikers have gone without food for three months. The *Guinness Book of World Records* carries the story of a man who, under medical supervision, fasted for more than a year. The purpose of his fast was to shed several hundred of the six hundred or so pounds of overweight he was carrying.

Generally speaking, a therapeutic fast -- even the short fast of one or two days, which you may undertake on your own -- leaves the body-mind ensemble healthier and better able to cope with the stresses of living. Some of the more specific benefits of the therapeutic fast are:

1. A loss of weight.
2. A saving of energy. The digestion of food requires a lot of energy. After a big meal one may become so drowsy as to fall asleep. Not having to digest food, the body saves energy, which can be put to use elsewhere. So, far from weakening you, fasting leaves you more energetic. Some long-distance runners of international caliber prepare themselves for major races by fasting for several days. Some of the very best enter the marathon, that most grueling of all running events, after a fast of two or more days; and, though they do not eat at all before the race, they do not falter during the race.

3. A biological house cleaning. Waste matter accumulates in the body from various sources -- the regular processing of food, the break-down of tissues through normal wear and tear, the inundation of our bodies' ecology by toxic substances from polluted food, water and air. Not having to cope with the processing of food and not having to clean up the mess that results from it, the body can get to work ridding itself of waste matter which it is often too busy to attend to.

4. A general overhaul. Daily, hourly, the body has to repair cells that break down or are destroyed by accidental injury. Frequently it is kept so busy processing unnecessarily big quantities of food and dealing with the poisons of caffeine and nicotine that it can look after only the most pressing repairs. A fast gives it a chance to catch up on overdue chores of maintenance. And, interestingly, during a fast, when the body gets no building materials from food, it uses re-cycled materials -- tissues worn out or diseased that have to be taken down.

Even one fast is usually enough to convince the novice that it is worthwhile to fast. You, too, owe it to yourself to read up on the benefits of fasting and to try at least one 24-hour "therapeutic" fast; for, the way you feel after even so short a fast will do more than anything I can say to prove to you that fasting makes sense.

Strategy 7: *a positive outlook* Few people realize how much the thoughts we entertain influence us -- our views, our expectations, our moods, our health, our whole lives. Think positive and you'll feel positive about yourself and your universe; permit yourself to think negative thoughts and everything about you is bound to assume a negative hue. We tend to think of our thoughts as something insubstantial, evanescent: they come, we entertain them for a while, and then they vanish as though they had never been. But that is not so. Our thoughts are a form of energy, which affects us and the world around us in very substantial ways: they can make us ill and they can make us well; they can make us miserable and they can make us happy; they can make us fail and they can make us succeed; they can, if employed the right way, "move mountains."

What we commonly regard as thoughts -- the thought processes that occur in our conscious minds -- is but a small part of them. Their roots reach deep into another part of us, elusive but very real. People call it by such names as the **subconscious**, the **unconscious**, the **spirit**, . No matter the name, it is the part where the real power of our thoughts lodges.

All too many people make their unconscious work against them rather than for them. The unconscious does not itself take sides for or against us. It simply notes our thoughts, good or bad, and acts on them. If we permit ourselves to think negative thoughts, whether we really mean them or not, the unconscious acts on them with the same dispassionate obedience as on positive thoughts. It matters little that they should be against our own best interests. Suppose there is a job I would like to get but I keep thinking, "Hopeless... lots of people much better than I are after the job ... no chance of me getting it" -- regardless whether I mean these thoughts, my unconscious takes note of them and gets to work on making this pessimistic projection of mine come true, sometimes in the most unexpected ways. It may, for instance, make me oversleep the morning of the interview. Had I thought optimistic thoughts, it would have got to work on making these thoughts come true.

Many years ago, an old Lincolnshire farmer, who overheard me exclaim, "How could I be so stupid!" after I had done something or other badly, took me aside and gently reprimanded me: "Don't do to yourself what you would not willingly take from another man. If you call yourself stupid every time you do something badly, you will end up believing that you are stupid." I did not understand till much later how wise the old man's counsel was.

In medical nomenclature, there is a term ***psychosomatic illness***, which refers to illness that has no basis in the corporeal parts of a patient but is believed to be brought about by his mind. Such illness can be every bit as real as any organic illness. A headache, asthma, allergies, eczema, diarrhea, high blood pressure, arthritis -- any of them and more can be and have been attributed to psychosomatic causes. Our thoughts can indeed make us ill.

That they can also make us well is most strikingly illustrated in the so-called placebo effect. A placebo is a substance which, though it has no known curative properties, effects a cure or at least an improvement in a patient's condition simply because the patient believes it has curative properties. Those patients who get well or a least better thanks to the placebo effect run into the millions. In fact, there are medical men who believe that many of the drugs used in Western Medicine -- supposedly real ones, not placebos -- owe much of their effectiveness to the placebo effect.

In a general sort of way, we can make our unconscious work <u>for</u> us rather than against us simply by banning negative thoughts from our minds and entertaining in their stead thoughts positive -- thoughts of health rather than thoughts of disease, thoughts of success rather than thoughts of failure, thoughts of optimism rather than thoughts of despair. We can, however, make our unconscious work for us in more specific ways. We can ask it to fulfil specific wishes for us. All we have to do is learn to communicate our wishes to the unconscious the right way. If we do, the unconscious will deliver....

Communicating wishes to the unconscious the right way means, above all, "sneaking" them past the watchdogs that guard the gates to the unconscious. A bit like trying to get a request to the boss. You know that the boss would say "yes" if only you could bring your request to his attention. The problem is getting it past the dragon of a secretary, who guards the approaches to his office. Now, the watchdogs at the gates of the unconscious never go away, but there are times when they relax their watchfulness. They do so when the conscious mind goes to sleep. But then you are asleep too and you can't transmit any wishes to the unconscious. Fortunately there are moments when the guardian dogs relax their watchfulness enough to let your request pass while you are still conscious enough to take advantage of the situation. I have in mind those magic moments that occur between waking and sleeping, morning and evening: the sharp dividing line between reality and dream begins to blur but you are still conscious enough to transmit a message which you thought out and formulated earlier, while fully awake.

    Here is how to go about it. You have gone to bed. The lights are out. You have closed your eyes. Now lie on your back and wriggle yourself into the most comfortable position you can find. Relax. If you wish, you may go through the relaxation routine ("Variation 4") on page 85. Otherwise just take a deep breath slowly and as slowly exhale. Then start "talking" to your unconscious -- talk as though you were talking to a real person. I actually address my unconscious as my **unconscious partner**.

    "Partner," I say, I need your help. "There is that ..., which I want so much but can see no way of getting. Help me...."
Then -- and this is probably the most important part of the transmission -- I visualize the object of my desire and project it on my inner screen. I hold it there for a little while, perhaps for a minute or two. I take delight in seeing it there, already come true. I do this morning and evening for a few days. I keep going back to the same picture but, where possible, I try to improve it. Then I "let go." I forget about it, confident that my

unconscious partner will do the rest. And (s)he usually does, often in the most surprising ways.

The whole procedure need not take more than five minutes. Don't worry if some evening you fall asleep before you finish your little act, or if some morning you forget, not to remember till you are up and away. Don't worry either if you find it difficult to believe in this sort of thing. It helps if you believe in what you are doing because you tend to do better what you believe in. But it works even if you do not believe in it, provided you take the transmission of your wish(es) seriously.

Let me give you an illustration from my own experience -- the story of how my unconscious partner got me to Africa some thirty years ago. I had done a lot of travelling in Europe and in North America. I had long wanted to go to Africa but had seen no way of doing so except as a tourist, something I had considered many times and rejected. I did not want to spend several thousand dollars for only a few weeks there. A few weeks would only whet my appetite, not appease the hunger. I wanted to spend a lot of time there, but there was no way I could afford to do so -- no way I could think of.

So I appealed to my unconscious partner, and (s)he came up with the ideal solution to the problem. One morning, while driving to some place or other, a sudden impulse prompted me to turn on the car radio, something I don't do very often. But that morning I did, quite accidentally, it seemed. And the first thing I heard, after the radio had crackled into operation, was that a group of people was in town recruiting teachers of English for Nigeria. I knew with instant certainty that that was for me. And it was. I went for an interview that same day, and three months later I was in Africa teaching English at the Borno College of Education in Maiduguri, north-eastern Nigeria. Accident, that I happened to turn on the radio at just the right time? You may think so; I don't. There have been too many of these apparent accidents in my life. I am convinced that it was my unconscious partner's doing.

You can enlist your unconscious partner's help with any problem. Trouble finding the right kind of job, trouble finding a partner in business, a health problem -- just ask your unconscious partner to help; (s)he will get you to the right place at the right time, (s)he will get you the information you need.

Say you have a health problem, which your doctor has not been able to solve or even to diagnose correctly. All you have to do is present the problem to your unconscious partner. Visualize the diseased part as cured and get out of the way. Your partner will do the rest. Two things are likely to happen. Your unconscious partner will mobilize the healing powers of your own body and (s)he will look for outside help if that is necessary. In the most unexpected ways, the most surprising ways, (s)he will nudge you to do the right thing. By apparent accident you pick up a magazine that contains some information about the very problem you are troubled with. By apparent accident you happen to meet someone who has experienced the same problem and who can give you valuable advice.

If negative thoughts are destructive, so are negative emotions. We cannot afford to let negative emotions dominate our lives. Envy, intolerance, anger, hate -- we cannot afford to indulge in these negative emotions. They drain us of psychic energy. They boomerang, hurting us more than the people they are aimed at. Positive emotions, on the other hand -- good will, tolerance, sympathy and love -- conserve, nay replenish our reserves of psychic energy. Confront people in anger and you come away drained. Meet them with love and you come away recharged. In three decades of teaching, I met many "angry teachers." They made life unnecessarily difficult for themselves. Anger in the teacher generates hostility in the students, and it takes so much more psychic energy to handle a crew of hostile students than one of students who are friendly and cooperative. The angry teachers are the ones who burn out prematurely.

Evidence is accumulating that there is a close correlation between negative emotions and illness, particularly cancer. People who are pessimistic in outlook, people who are tense with hatred or anger are much more likely to come down with cancer than people who yield to love and are optimistic. Which side are you going to be on? Better learn to eradicate negative habits of thought and feeling and to cultivate positive ones instead.

There must be a balance. The various parts of a human being -- body, mind, soul -- are parts only because we have arbitrarily chosen to segment the whole. Our having separate names for them does not mean that they exist separately. They form a whole, and what happens to one affects the others.

A few pages back, I talked about the fact that our thoughts and our emotions can bring about physical illness. By the same token, things that appear to be of the body only can bring about mental illness. Faulty nutrition can affect mental health. Take the B-vitamins. A deficiency in almost any of them can cause serious mental disturbances, some of them indistinguishable from schizophrenia. A sluggish vascular system, the wages of lack of exercise, results in poor oxygenation of the billions of cells that make up the human body. Brain cells are among the first to be affected. And, if brain cells do not function optimally, mind -- whatever it is -- cannot function optimally either. For mind does not exist in isolation. It is a function of the nervous system. I would go a step further. What I have been calling the unconscious partner -- call it spirit, if you wish -- is also connected with and dependent on the nervous system. It is that fragment of eternity in each one of us, through which we are in touch with our universe. But, if it has to operate through a nervous system impaired through faulty nutrition, a nervous system slowed owing to poor oxygenation, a nervous system dulled by liquor, nicotine or other drugs -- it is itself bound to be out of tune. It is not capable of receiving the faint signals which arrive from who knows where -- sudden hunches, premonitions, urges that nudge us to the right place at the right time.

When viewed in this light, good health transcends the level of mere physical and mental well-being. It becomes a moral issue. Unless I keep myself in the best possible state of heath, communication between me and God suffers. He prays best who is healthiest.

Positive thoughts then, and positive emotions -- these are two of the elements of a positive outlook. A third one is faith. Have faith in your body, its ability to take care of itself. Have faith in your ability to make a difference by practicing the seven strategies of healthful living. Have faith in your ability to make a difference by practicing positive habits of thought and feeling. It comes free of charge and it is not difficult.

V

NOTHING TO LOSE BUT MUCH TO GAIN

Most people regard illness as something inevitable, something that is bound to strike everyone sooner or later. Whether it strikes a particular individual sooner or later they think is largely a matter of genetic accident according as (s)he is endowed with more or less natural resistance to disease. And most people regard loss of health as one of the worst things -- if not the worst -- that can happen to them. Some spend fortunes in attempts, often futile, to regain lost health. Now, if they learned of some form of magic guaranteed to make them healthy and to keep them healthy far into old age, what would they not give for it! But that magic does exist, and it is for everyone, rich and poor. It is free of charge. That magic is the naturopathic way of living set out in Chapter III.

In Chapter II, we looked at the limitations of Western Medicine. There I tried to demonstrate that Western Medicine is far from having all the answers and that, above all, it does not generate health. I also pointed out that genuinely healthy people -- individuals, or groups such as the Hunza -- owe their good health to a healthful lifestyle, not to the ministrations of Western Medicine. They are the ones who, by and large, do *not* consume drugs. It is the sick who do, and often the drugs make them sicker.

An alternative system of health care, Naturopathic Medicine, was presented in Chapter III. Some fundamental differences between Western Medicine and Naturopathy were pointed out, the most important one being the fact that the latter puts the responsibility for health squarely on the shoulders of the individual while the former arrogates all responsibility and all competence to itself. The latter maintains that a healthful way of living will do more for a person's health than all the ministrations of Western Medicine. To the former this is anathema. It is dangerous fadism and quackery. Western Medicine wants patients who are uninformed and leave everything to the doctor: Naturopathy regards as the ideal patient one who is generally well informed, knows how to take care of his own health and is willing to do so.

Taking care of one's health means, primarily, practicing the seven strategies of healthful living, which I discussed in some detail in Chapter IV. Anyone who practices them reasonably conscientiously will be richly rewarded. He will enjoy lasting good health. He will be liberated from the insidious fear, which overshadows the lives of the majority of human beings -- the fear of sickness. Just think of it! No more sick days in bed, no more visits to doctors' offices, no more admissions to hospital. Wouldn't it be wonderful!

Good health will moreover mean big savings in terms of money not spent on medical services or drugs, in terms of workdays not lost to illness. Good health will mean more time and more energy to meet the demands of life. Good health will ultimately mean a greater potential for happiness.

If this health magic is to be practiced widely, governments have to get into the act. First and foremost they must initiate changes in medical orientation -- a shift of emphasis from corrective to genuinely preventive medicine. It will mean training a new breed of medical doctors, who believe that most illness can be prevented through a healthful lifestyle and who can and will teach their patients what a healthful lifestyle means.

Governments must see to it that the great army of ordinary people is educated and/or re-educated 1) to understand the benefits of good health, 2) to understand that they themselves are responsible for their health, and 3) to understand how best to go about building and maintaining health.

Governments must do more. They must put a ban on the refining of food, especially of grain. Such a step would result in tremendous savings both in terms of the quantity of available food resources and in terms of their nutritional quality.

And governments must shift their emphasis from buying drugs to buying supplements -- vitamins and minerals to build health rather than drugs that do no more than treat the symptoms of disease. The prices of supplements should, and could, be kept low so that even ordinary people can afford to buy them

The rewards of shifting from a system of health care based on Western Medicine to one based on Naturopathy would be immense. It would, if nothing else, solve the seemingly unsolvable problem of rising health care costs. As it is, most countries in the world, even the richest of developed countries, are finding it more and more difficult to pay their health care bills. West Germany, one of the very richest countries in the world, is a case in point.

A shift to Naturopathy would mean savings in other areas too. A population of healthy people would lose few days of work due to sickness. The savings there would be incalculable. And genuinely healthy people would be more productive in every line of work.

A population of healthy people would be happier than one of predominantly sick people. A society of such people would be a better place to live in. So why not try? There is nothing to lose, but lots to gain. Of course many doctors would have to re-think their jobs and a good many of them would lose their jobs. Moreover, the profits of Big Pharma and of the makers of medical gear would go down. But surely we don't want to keep vast armies of people sick so as to keep doctors employed and to guaranty big dividends for the pharma-industry. Let's have real HEALTH, not just HEALTH CARE, for all....

VI

Appendix

Possible alternative treatments for

common problems

The intent of this appendix is to give you a few hints regarding relevant web searches. Inform yourself before you gullibly swallow pills which may make you sicker. For example, do a web search for "baking soda and cancer." Just be careful to separate the wheat from the chaff when you look at the results. At any rate, the things I suggest below are things I would at least investigate.

For a heart-warming story, search for and read "Vernon's Dance With Cancer." You can just search for the title itself or you can access the story here: <http://phkillscancer.com/vernons_dance_with_cancer.

Alzheimer's	coconut oil, 3 T a day, plus turmeric, 1 t in warm water twice a day
Arthritis	magnesium, a precursor of hyaluronic acid… hyaluronic acid by itself… niacinamide… cinnamon and honey…vegetable juices
Asthma	whey shakes and antioxidants… Pantothenic acid (a B vitamin)
Hypertension	garlic, cayenne, celery juice, regular aerobic exercise, a predominantly vegetarian diet
Cancer	baking soda… celery juice… both tend to raise the pH above 7; if the pH is raised to values above 8, the cancer cells have no chance… extra vitamin D… a vegetarian diet of raw food… B6… oral iodine… selenium
Diabetes	a vegetarian diet of raw food… it's the enzymes that make all the Difference… flavonoids –

	tea, resveratrol, silymarin, cinnamon extract, quercetin, and urcumin… Vitamin E
Influenza	Vitamin D (2000 IU in summer, 5000 in winter)… a daily 3000 to 5000 mg of C to prevent the flu, more to cure it
Heart disease	cayenne… 1 t in warm water drunk twice a day… cinnamon and honey
MS	coconut oil… Vitamin D
Parkinson's	coconut oil… Vitamin D
Sinus	cinnamon and honey… salt water irrigation

VII

Bibliography

1. Abrahamson, E.B. and Prezet, A.W. BODY

MIND AND SUGAR. Pyramid Books, New York, 1973.

2. Airola, Paavo, Ph. D. ARE YOU CONFUSED? Health Plus Publishers, Phoenix, Arizona,1977.

3. Atkins, M.D. DR. ATKINS DIETREVOLUTION. Bantam Books, New York, 1973.

4. Bieler, Henry G. FOOD IS YOUR BEST MEDICINE. Vintage Books, New York, 1973.

5. Blech, Joerg. DIE KRANKHEITSERFINDER. (The Disease inventors). S. Fischer Verlag, Frankfurt, 2004.

6. Bloomfield, H.H., M.D., et. al. TM: DISCOVERING INNER ENERGY AND OVERCOMING STRESS. Dell Publishing Co., New York, 1975.

7. Clark, Linda. KNOW YOUR NUTRITION. Keats Publishing, New Canaan, Connecticut, 1973.

8. Cooper, Kenneth H., M.D. AEROBICS. Bantam Books, New York, 1972.

9. Cooper, Mildred and Cooper, Kenneth H., M.D. AEROBICS FOR WOMEN. Bantam Books, New York, 1972.

10. Cott, Allan, M.D. FASTING AS A WAY OF LIFE. Bantam Books, New York, 1977.

11. Cott, Allan, M.D. FASTING: THE ULTIMATE DIET. Bantam Books, New York, 1975.

12. Dufty, William. SUGAR BLUES.Warner Books, New York,1975.

13. Elwood, Catharyn. FEEL LIKE A MILLION. Pocket Books, New York, 1972.

14. Erasmus, Udo, Ph.D. FATS AND OILS. Alive Books, Vancouver, B.C., 1986.

15. Fredericks, Carlton, Ph.D. and Goodman Herman, M.D. LOW BLOOD SUGAR AND YOU. Constellation International, New York, 1973.

16. Hittleman, Richard. YOGA: 28 DAY EXERCISE PLAN. Workman Publishing Company, New York, 1969.

17. Langbein, Kurt et al. BITTERE PILLEN. (Nutzen und Risiken der Arzneimittel – BITTER PILLS, Usefulness and Risks of Medical Drugs) April 2005. (No English Translation)

18. LeShan, Lawrence. HOW TO MEDITATE Bantam Books, New York, 1975.

19. Mendelsohn, Robert S. MD CONFESSIONS OF A MEDICAL HERETIC. Amazon.com

20. Moore Lappe, Frances. DIET FOR A SMALL PLANET. Ballantine Books, New York, 1972.

21, Morehouse, Lawrence E., Ph. D. TOTAL ITNESS. Simon and Schuster, New York, 1975.

22. Pauling, Linus, Ph.D. HOW TO LIVE LONGER AND FEEL BETTER. W.H. Freeman & Co., N.Y., 1986.

23. Robin, Anthony. UNLIMITED POWER. Ballantine, 1986.

24. Shelton, Herbert M. FASTING CAN SAVE YOUR LIFE. Hygiene Press, Chicago, 1967.

25. Watts, Allan. MEDITATION. Celestial Arts, 231 Adrian Road, Millbrae, California, 1974.

26. Webb, Audry T. SLIMMING WITH YOGA. Simon and Schuster, New York, 1970.

27. Williams,Roger, Ph.D. NUTRTITION GAINST DISEASE. Bantam Books, New York, 1973.

Made in the USA
Lexington, KY
09 October 2015